Mother
&baby
EXERCISE

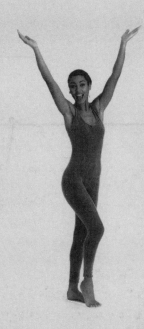

WARD LOCK

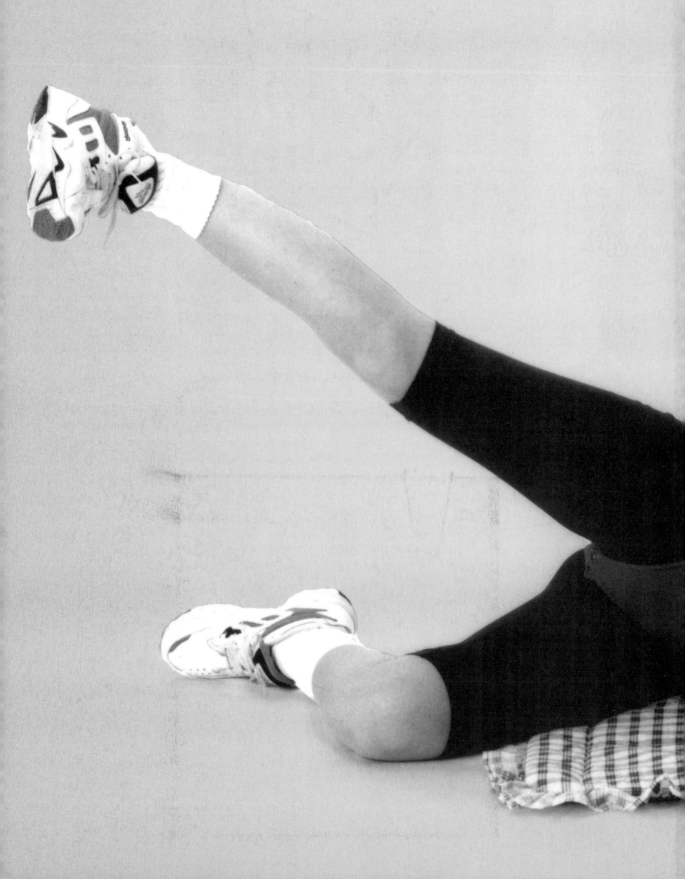

Mother
&baby
EXERCISE

An Easy Fitness Programme to take you through Pregnancy

— • —

EMMA SCATTERGOOD

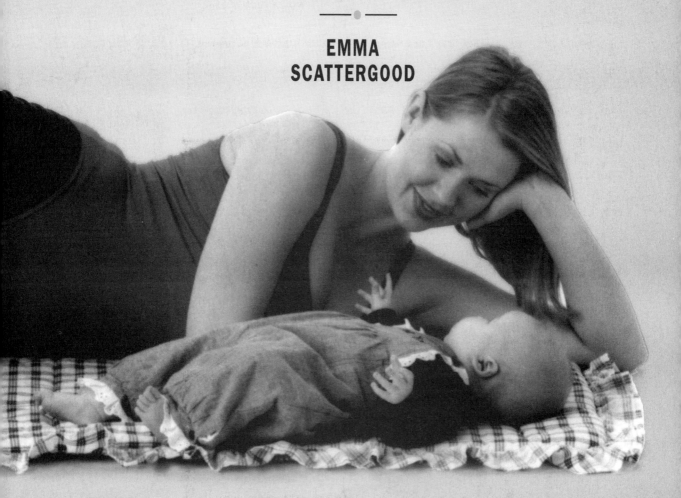

A WARD LOCK BOOK

First published in the UK 1995 by Ward Lock
Wellington House, 125 Strand
LONDON, WC2R 0BB
A Cassell Imprint

Distributed in the United States by Sterling Publishing Co., Inc.
387 Park Avenue South, New York, NY 10016-8810

Distributed in Australia by Capricorn Link (Australia) Pty Ltd
2/13 Carrington Road, Castle Hill NSW 2154

A British Library Cataloguing in Publication Data block for this book may be
obtained from the British Library

ISBN 0 7063 7392 8
Designed by Richard Carr
Typeset by Method Limited, Epping, Essex
Printed and bound in Great Britain

With thanks to the following for their help with the book:

Exercise Consultant: Judy Di Fiore, YMCA, London
Photographer: Steve Shott
Activity gym on page 122 courtesy of Early Learning Centre,
'Octopull' on page 123 courtesy of the Boots Company plc.

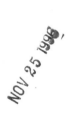

CONTENTS

INTRODUCTION

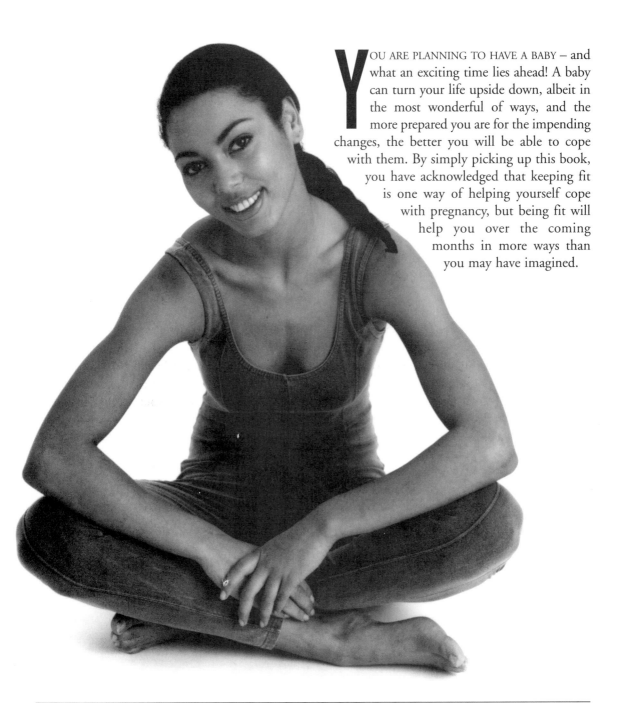

Y OU ARE PLANNING TO HAVE A BABY – and what an exciting time lies ahead! A baby can turn your life upside down, albeit in the most wonderful of ways, and the more prepared you are for the impending changes, the better you will be able to cope with them. By simply picking up this book, you have acknowledged that keeping fit is one way of helping yourself cope with pregnancy, but being fit will help you over the coming months in more ways than you may have imagined.

Why is keeping fit so important? Unromantic as it may be, it is useful to think of your body as a factory on the brink of manufacturing a wonderful new product: unless every part of the factory is working smoothly and doing the best job that it can, there will be some hiccups in the production process, and the finished product may not even be quite as good as it could have been. Ideally, the factory should be cleaned up, and any problems smoothed out well in advance, so that the whole operation is working perfectly before production even begins. So, the healthier and fitter you are, the more likely you are to become pregnant quickly, the better your body will cope with the stresses and strains of pregnancy, and the healthier your baby will be, too.

What does keeping fit entail? It certainly does not mean you have to turn into some sort of marathon runner – being fit does not mean being superwoman. It simply means that your body stays healthy and strong enough to cope with the combined rigours of pregnancy and everyday living – and that you will have even more energy for leisure activities.

Getting fit need not take much effort or time either. This book contains a series of workouts that need not take up more than 20 minutes every other day – so even the busiest of people can find time to do them – and they do not involve jumping around! Yet, despite being short and simple, they will tone and strengthen your muscles, so that you look good and feel better. None of the workouts demand that you do, say, 20 press-ups at a time – although you can if you want to. You set your own level and increase the amount of work you do as and when you are ready.

Of course being fit is not just about having a healthy body: a healthy mind is essential too. Feeling worried can be just as damaging as a physical problem, so this book aims to help you overcome the difficulties common at this time, teaching you how to relax properly.

You are planning on starting or increasing your family, and no doubt already have hopes and aspirations for your children. You will want them to grow up happy and healthy, so why not start setting them a good example – before they are even born? Establish a pattern of healthy living now, and your children will soon be following your lead. The book even includes a 'workout' for your baby, so that he or she can enjoy the best possible start to a fit and healthy life. (The baby in our photographs is a girl, so we have referred to babies as 'she' throughout, although of course all the information and exercises apply equally to both sexes.) The workouts in this book are not simply for pregnancy, they can be for life – so why not start now?

CHAPTER ONE

THE WARM-UP

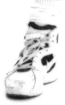

S O, YOU HAVE DECIDED it is time to start exercising. Before you leap into action and start any of the workouts, it is important to read this chapter and perform the warm-up exercises given here. These will help make your workout safer and more effective.

You will need to return to this chapter each time you work out, so take time to get the exercises right. Technique is extremely important. You may wish to record yourself reading the instructions out loud; then, once you have grasped what is required from the pictures, you can listen to your tape instead.

THE PELVIC FLOOR: MUSCLES YOU NEVER KNEW YOU HAD

As soon as you become pregnant you will hear a lot of talk about 'pelvic floor' muscles. You will be asked to exercise them frequently throughout this book, so what are they and why are they so important?

The pelvic floor muscles lie in the base of your pelvis, between and surrounding the anus, urethra and vagina, and are a vital support for the contents of your abdomen and pelvis. We should all be exercising them regularly, pregnant or not, to prevent embarrassing leaks of urine whenever we laugh, sneeze or lift something, but when you become pregnant, the hormones that make your joints and ligaments soft also soften the pelvic floor, so these muscles need even more attention than normal.

In the light of all this, you will be reminded to exercise your pelvic floor in every workout in this book. However, it is never too early to start, so try the exercise now.

At first, you may find it hard even to locate exactly where the pelvic floor muscles are. To help pinpoint them, some women imagine they are trying to stop themselves from passing urine, or are holding in a tampon. Try stopping your flow of urine next time you go to the toilet (do not forget to allow the urine to continue on its course once you have released the muscles, or you may get an infection). Once you have found the muscles, you can exercise them anywhere and any time, although you may find some positions easier than others.

The exercise

Tighten your pelvic floor muscles and draw them upwards, starting with the area around the back passage and moving gradually towards the front. Hold for a count of four and then slowly let go. Try to repeat this five times.

Next, imagine you are in a lift and, instead of shooting straight to the top floor, make several stops as you pull the muscles upwards. When you release, make several stops on the way down too. Try to repeat this five times.

Do several sets of these exercises a day – perhaps each time you make a cup of tea. And, if you still feel lacking in incentive, remember that strong pelvic floor muscles can do wonders for your sex life, too!

POSTURE CHECK

Over the nine months of your pregnancy, your body will be changing constantly and will be put under increasing pressure. By maintaining a good posture, you can reduce the strain on your back and joints – and you will look better, too!

A lot of pregnant women forget about good posture and adopt the 'pregnant slouch', sticking their bump out in front and developing an exaggerated lower back curve (see overleaf). The following routine should prevent that happening. Practise now: it is important to maintain good posture whenever you are exercising.

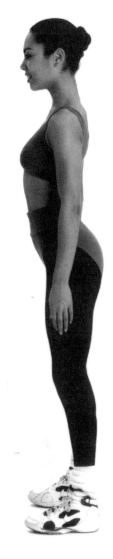

Bad

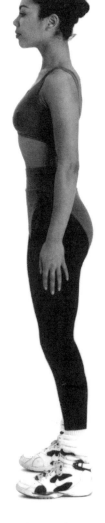

Good

1 Stand with your feet hip-width apart and keep your knees directly over your ankles. Relax your knees slightly.

2 Gently shift your upper body backwards and forwards until you find the point where you feel most evenly balanced.

3 Tilt your pelvis forwards and slightly upwards, to tuck your bottom under and lift your bump (when you have one!) upwards. Pull

in your abdominal muscles to support your baby. This reduces the stress on your lower back and is called the 'pelvic tilt'.

4 Bring your shoulders back slightly so that your chest opens, and then bring them down to lengthen your neck.

5 Lift your ribcage out of your waist and grow tall, lengthening your spine and lifting the top of your head higher towards the ceiling.

Health and safety

- If you have had previous miscarriages, back or joint problems, seek the advice of your doctor BEFORE you start exercising.

- Never exercise if you feel any pain in your back or strain on your pelvic floor muscles.

- Wear comfortable clothing which allows you to move freely.

- For any activity that involves jogging or jumping, you should wear supportive training shoes. It is fine to wear trainers for the workouts in this book, but bare feet are sufficient.

- Never exercise in just socks or tights, as you may slip.

- Read the instructions for each exercise carefully before you begin.

- Make sure you start each one in a good position.

- Maintain good posture throughout.

- Breathe freely.

- Avoid making any jerking or bouncing movements.

- Stay in control of your body's movements.

- Maintain a regular rhythm.

- Listen to your body: do not push yourself if you become short of breath or tired.

- Stop IMMEDIATELY if you feel any pain (especially in your back or legs), nausea, dizziness or have difficulty in walking.

- Go to hospital if you have any vaginal bleeding or your waters break.

- NEVER skip the warm-up or cool down. It is important to stretch your muscles before and after exercise or you could risk damaging them.

THE WARM-UP

This warm-up should be used throughout your pregnancy before you start any of the routines in this book. Do NOT skip it! However, as your pregnancy progresses, you may wish to adapt some parts slightly, so follow the notes in the relevant chapters. On days when you are not feeling very energetic, you can always just do the warm-up routine for a simple stretch workout.

You will need a stable chair with a high back for support for some exercises, so have one ready.

1 POSTURE CHECK
Stand (or sit), paying attention to your posture and looking straight ahead.

2 SHOULDER LIFTS
Looking straight ahead, lift your right shoulder up towards your right ear and gently lower it again. Repeat on the other side. Then repeat the sequence five times.

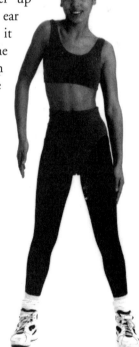

3 SHOULDER ROLLS

Lift both your shoulders and roll them forwards, five times.

Lift both shoulders up again and press them gently back and down to open your chest. Repeat five times.

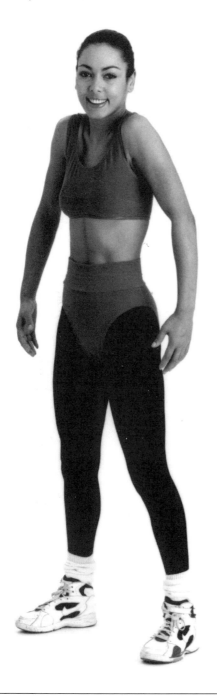

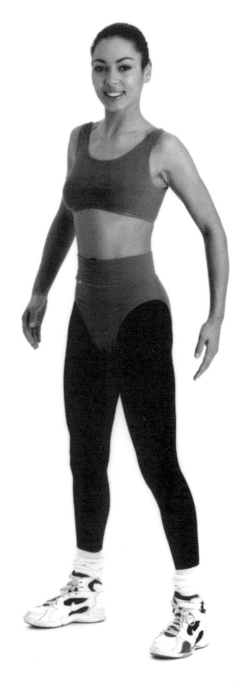

4 NECK MOBILITY

Move your right ear slowly to your right shoulder, then return to the centre. Repeat slowly to the left, then return to the centre. Repeat five times.

Bring your chin down towards your chest, then return to the centre. Repeat five times.

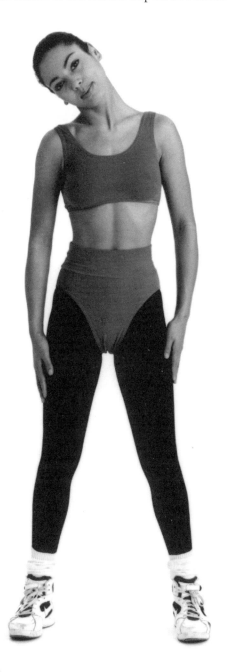

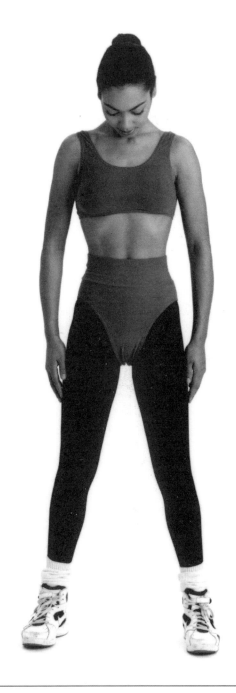

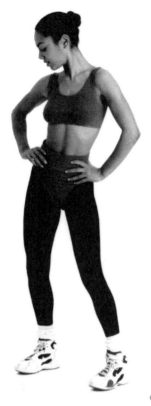

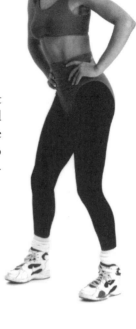

5 HIP CIRCLES

This mobilizes your spine. Put your hands on your hips and gently move your hips to the right, forwards, then left. Aim to make one fluid, circular movement. Repeat five times.

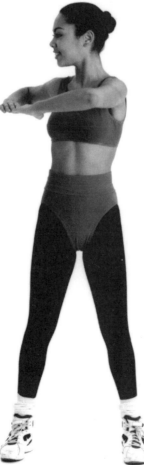

6 WAIST TWISTS

Bring your elbows out at shoulder level and twist slowly at the waist round to the left. Return to the centre, and twist to the right. Repeat five times.

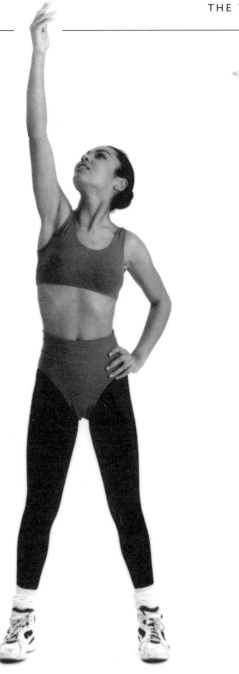

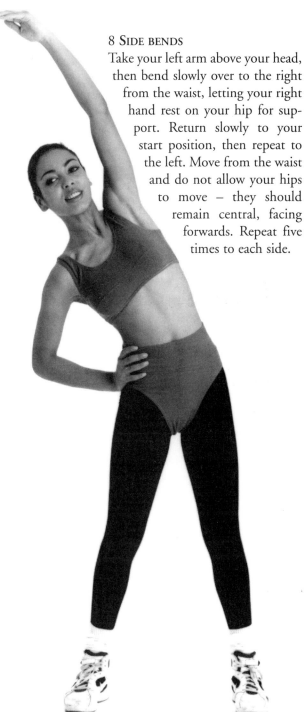

8 SIDE BENDS
Take your left arm above your head, then bend slowly over to the right from the waist, letting your right hand rest on your hip for support. Return slowly to your start position, then repeat to the left. Move from the waist and do not allow your hips to move – they should remain central, facing forwards. Repeat five times to each side.

7 UPWARD REACH
Slowly lift one arm straight up towards the ceiling and stretch up high out of your waist. Repeat with the other arm. Repeat five times with each arm, keeping the other hand on your hip.

9 KNEE BENDS

Check your posture. With your hands gently resting at the top of your thighs, and your feet a little more than hip-distance apart, slowly bend your knees so that they come out over your toes. Then return slowly to your start position. Do not bend too far. Make sure that you maintain a pelvic tilt while you do this and keep your tummy muscles tight, so that your back remains straight and you do not stick your bottom out. Repeat five times.

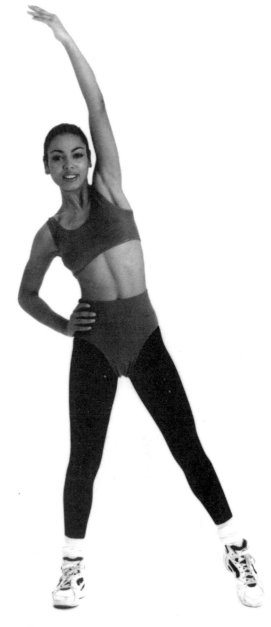

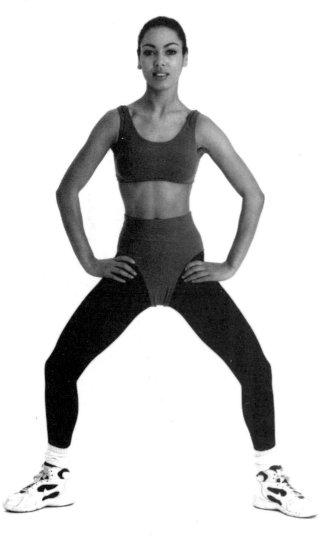

10 SWAY AND STRETCH

Repeat the knee bends, but this time, as you come up, reach your left arm up high towards the ceiling and slightly over to the right, lifting your left heel off the floor as you do so. Repeat to the other side. Then repeat the sequence, moving from left to right, five times.

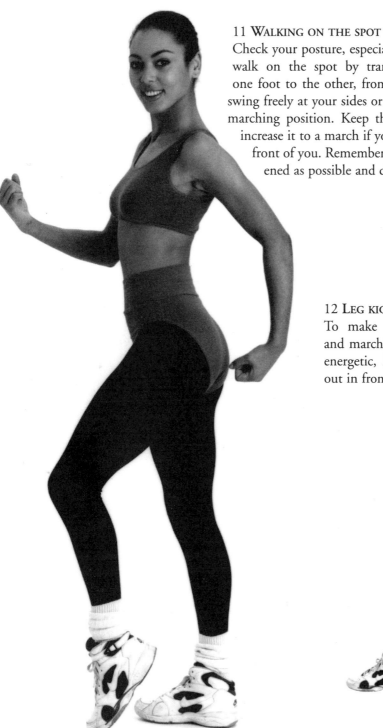

11 WALKING ON THE SPOT

Check your posture, especially your pelvic tilt, and then walk on the spot by transferring your weight from one foot to the other, from toe to heel. Let your arms swing freely at your sides or bring them up into a strong marching position. Keep the pace steady at first, then increase it to a march if you wish, lifting your knees in front of you. Remember to keep your back as lengthened as possible and do not sink into your hips.

12 LEG KICKS

To make your walking and marching a bit more energetic, kick your legs out in front of you.

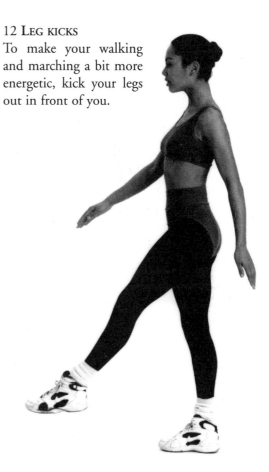

13 ANKLE CIRCLES

Using a wall or a stable chair for support, bring one leg forward or out to the side and circle the ankle round to the left, then round to the right. Repeat with the other leg, really making the ankle work.

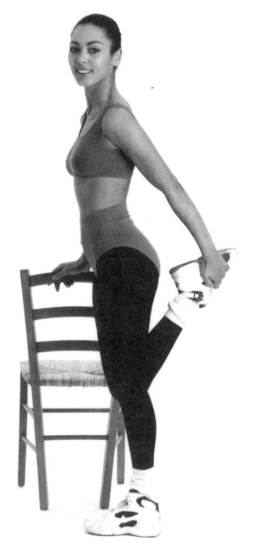

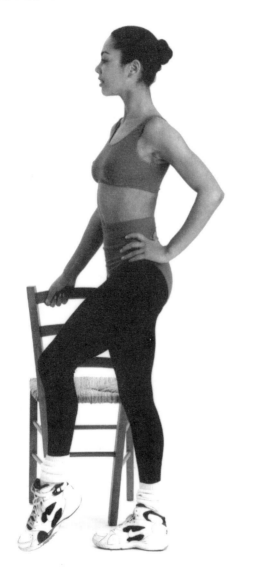

14 QUADRICEP STRETCH

Stand well, with a pelvic tilt, holding on to the back of a chair for support. Bring one foot up behind you and, holding on to your toes, bring it up close towards your bottom. Stand as upright as you can (check your pelvic tilt once more) and bend your supporting leg a little. Hold it for a count of four to feel the stretch at the front of your thigh. Release slowly and repeat with your other leg. Stop if you feel any pain in or around your knees.

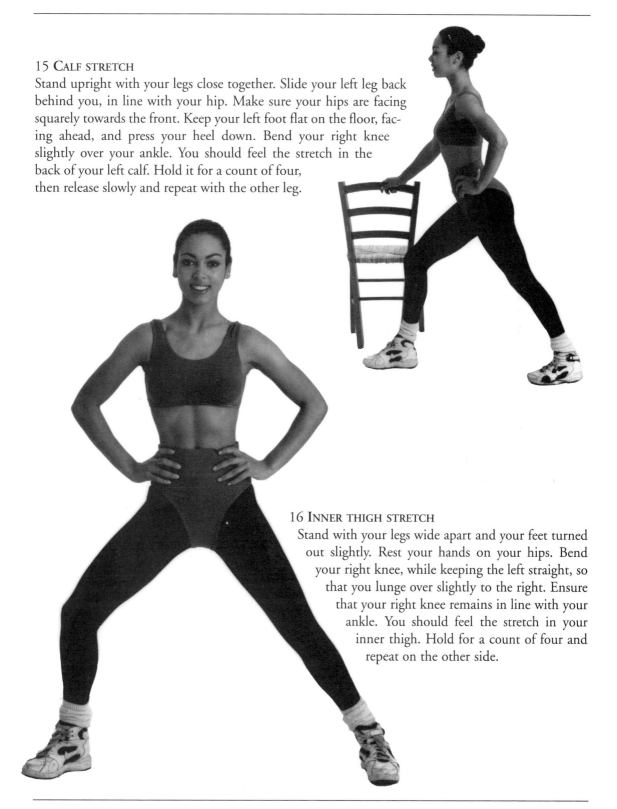

15 CALF STRETCH

Stand upright with your legs close together. Slide your left leg back behind you, in line with your hip. Make sure your hips are facing squarely towards the front. Keep your left foot flat on the floor, facing ahead, and press your heel down. Bend your right knee slightly over your ankle. You should feel the stretch in the back of your left calf. Hold it for a count of four, then release slowly and repeat with the other leg.

16 INNER THIGH STRETCH

Stand with your legs wide apart and your feet turned out slightly. Rest your hands on your hips. Bend your right knee, while keeping the left straight, so that you lunge over slightly to the right. Ensure that your right knee remains in line with your ankle. You should feel the stretch in your inner thigh. Hold for a count of four and repeat on the other side.

17 PECTORAL STRETCH

Standing upright, take both arms right behind your back and, with your hands held loosely together, push your arms straight back to push your chest open. Hold for a count of four.

18 TRAPEZIUS STRETCH

Now take your arms in front of you and stretch your shoulders forwards as far as you can, while keeping your back upright. Feel the stretch across your upper back. Hold for a count of four.

19 TRICEP STRETCH

Take your left arm behind your head, bending at the elbow. Use your right hand on the left elbow to ease the left arm gently down behind your head. Then change arms to stretch the right tricep.

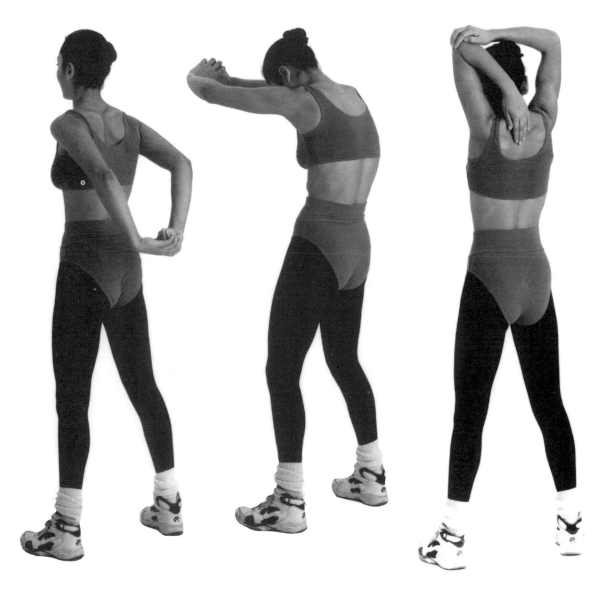

Your muscle groups

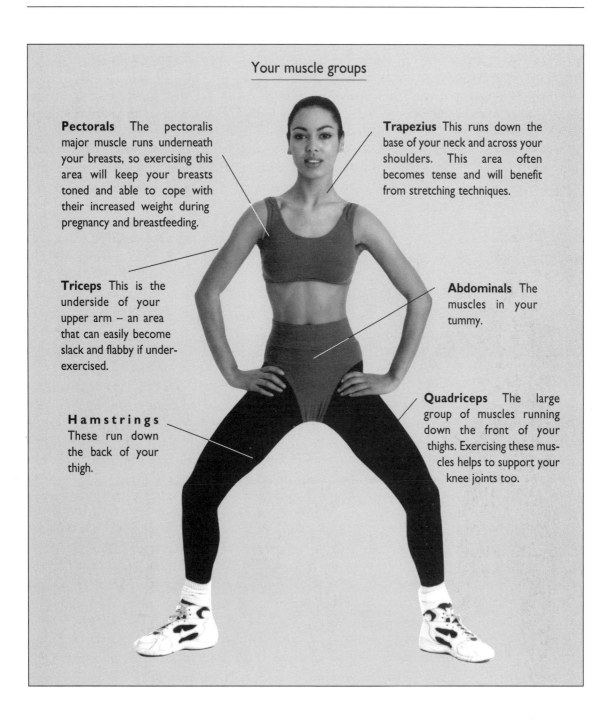

Pectorals The pectoralis major muscle runs underneath your breasts, so exercising this area will keep your breasts toned and able to cope with their increased weight during pregnancy and breastfeeding.

Trapezius This runs down the base of your neck and across your shoulders. This area often becomes tense and will benefit from stretching techniques.

Triceps This is the underside of your upper arm – an area that can easily become slack and flabby if under-exercised.

Abdominals The muscles in your tummy.

Hamstrings These run down the back of your thigh.

Quadriceps The large group of muscles running down the front of your thighs. Exercising these muscles helps to support your knee joints too.

NOW you are ready to start your workouts – good luck!

CHAPTER TWO

GETTING FIT FOR PREGNANCY

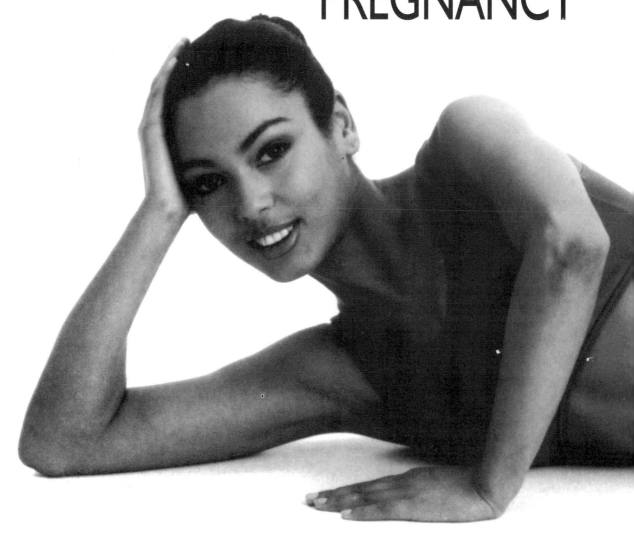

SOME OF YOU MAY BE SURPRISED to see this chapter here at all. Why bother changing the way you treat your body *before* you conceive – after all, it is not going to affect the baby, is it?

Well, the answer is, it does. Not only that, but it can make a big difference to how you cope with the pregnancy and birth. So, for the sake of your baby – and yourself – it is time to reassess the way you live and make a few changes.

STEP ONE: START EXERCISING

Perhaps it is hardly surprising that this is top of the list – keeping fit is what this book is about, after all.

But exercise really can make a big difference to you, your partner and your baby: a baby's health has been shown to depend very much on the health of its mother *and* father before and at the time of conception. If you are both fit and well, you stand a greater chance of conceiving, continuing the pregnancy to term (the baby's due date), and having a healthy baby.

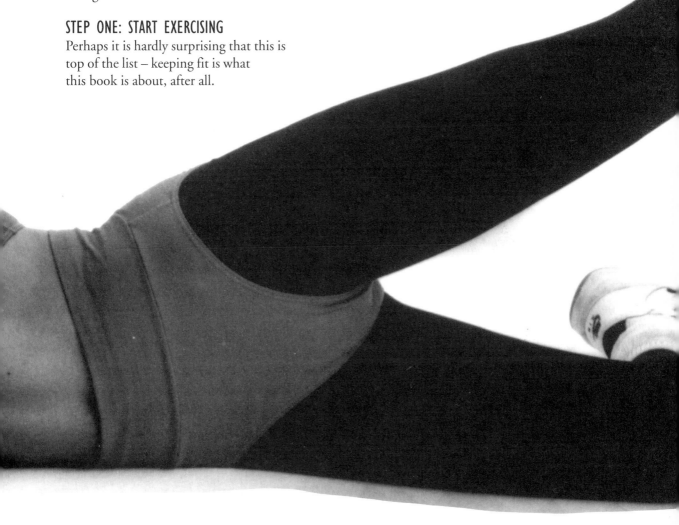

Pregnancy will also put an extra strain on your joints and ligaments, so the fitter you are, and the stronger your body, the better you will be able to cope. In fact most women who exercise up to conception and during their pregnancy find that not only do they look firmer and better than those who do not, they also suffer far less from the common pregnancy niggles such as backache, constipation and so on. Exercise has also been shown to give you an emotional lift, due to the hormones it releases in your body, so you really will feel better for doing it.

If all this still has not quite convinced you to leap into action, then consider just one more point: women who exercise before and during their pregnancy are also far more likely to snap back into shape after the baby is born. What an incentive!

How to start

What sort of exercise should you be doing? Until you actually become pregnant, you can do whatever exercise appeals to you in order to keep fit. After you conceive, you will have to take a little more care (see Chapter 3).

Until then you should aim for at least 20 minutes of aerobic exercise three times a week, combined with stretching exercises to start and finish (such as the ones in this book). An aerobic exercise is one that increases your pulse rate, making you breathe a little bit faster. Jogging, swimming, cycling and dancing are all ideal, but a brisk stroll is just as good, and a great way to get started. It is easy to fit into your normal routine and does not require any special exercise gear, just a good pair of low, supportive shoes.

The important thing is to choose a form of exercise you will stick to. A quick spurt of activity,

followed by a week or so of doing nothing at all, will not keep you fit. You need to do it regularly.

Begin at a gentle pace, slowly building up to one that feels right for you. If you do not overdo it, exercise should eventually give you more energy, not tire you out. Give yourself a day's rest between each session in order to let your muscles recover.

STEP TWO: STOP SMOKING

You may already be full of good intentions to stop when you actually become pregnant, but if either you or your partner smoke, you really should stop now. You already know that it is not good for your health, but did you know that it can also cause a low sperm count? So smoking will also reduce your chances of conceiving in the first place.

Once you are pregnant, it is imperative that you do not smoke or have a smoky atmosphere in your house, so that your baby is not forced to become a passive smoker. Smoking is associated with miscarriage, stillbirth, damage to the placenta, an increased risk of malformations and low birthweight babies. New research has also shown a link between smoking and cot death. And, looking ahead, if you continue to smoke as your baby grows up, he or she may not grow as they should and may even have learning difficulties.

So, kick the habit as soon as you can. Your doctor will be able to give you advice and put you in touch with local support groups.

STEP THREE: SWITCH TO SOFT DRINKS

A normal, healthy adult is advised to drink no more than 14 units of alcohol a week: that is 14 glasses of wine, or seven pints of beer. If you are planning on having a baby, though, you should cut right down, and preferably give up altogether, three months before conceiving. Alcohol damages a man's sperm and a woman's ovum, so your chances of conceiving are reduced if you are a drinker.

Once you become pregnant, a large intake of alcohol can lead to foetal alcohol syndrome, which results in retarded growth and mental ability, damage to the nervous system and brain, and even stillbirth.

It is difficult to set a 'safe' level of drinking during pregnancy, as alcohol affects everyone differently and some people can safely consume more than others. Ideally, you should give up completely in order to be sure that you are not putting your baby at risk – but the odd glass of wine is not going to hurt.

STEP FOUR: DROP THE DRUGS

Of course, we are not all hardened heroin addicts, but a lot of us take more painkillers than perhaps is necessary. From now on, only take over-the-counter medicines when it really is vital and tell your doctor that you are planning to conceive if he or she writes you a prescription for anything.

If you do take any 'social' drugs, cut them out now. Women are advised to avoid them for the sake of both their and their baby's health. A man's sperm count can also be affected by drugs and will take some months to recover. Hard drugs will also damage the chromosomes in his sperm, increasing the risk of your baby having some abnormality.

If you are on the pill at the moment, talk to your doctor about your plans to conceive. He or she will probably advise you to come off the pill about a month or two before you start trying for a baby (and use barrier methods in the meantime), so that you have one normal

Further checks

In order to be sure that you are fit to conceive, there are a few other checks worth making before you try to become pregnant.

• Book a smear test if you have not had one recently. All women should have one at least every three years, in order to check the cervix for cancerous cells. Do not panic if your smear is abnormal: problem cells detected early can be treated quickly and painlessly.

• Ask your doctor about your immunity to German Measles. You will probably have had a vaccination when you were younger, but the antibodies become less efficient as time goes on, so you may need another injection now. German Measles poses a serious risk to your baby if you catch it while you are pregnant, especially in the first three months, and it can cause malformations, such as blindness, deafness and heart disease.

• Check that you do not have any sexually transmitted diseases, and get them treated if you have. If you have herpes during pregnancy, and especially at the time of the birth, your baby could become infected too, and you may be advised to have a Caesarean section to reduce this risk.

menstrual period first. If you become pregnant while you are still on the pill, stop taking it immediately.

EATING FOR TWO?

Pregnancy is not an excuse to eat anything and everything! In fact, the phrase 'eating for two' is something you should forget straightaway –

double helpings are certainly not on the agenda. That said, pregnancy is certainly not a time for dieting either, so if you are slightly overweight and want to lose some pounds, do it now, before you conceive, and not afterwards.

What you should be doing already, and continuing once you are pregnant, is eating a healthy, balanced diet, with plenty of raw fruit and vegetables, fibre and protein. There will be stages in your pregnancy when you are hungrier than usual, but try to reach for something nutritious to nibble, rather than sugary or fatty snacks. Your baby's diet depends entirely on what you eat, so his birth weight and future health are influenced by your eating habits too.

There are no special diets for pregnancy. Just be sure to eat a good variety of foods, including some from each of the main food groups every day:

• Starchy foods, such as potatoes, bread and cereals.

• Fresh fruit and vegetables.

• Lean meat, poultry, oily fish or a vegetarian alternative, such as nuts and beans.

• Low-fat dairy foods.

There are some foods you should avoid during pregnancy, however (see Chapter 3).

As long as you eat well now and during pregnancy, you should not need to take any extra vitamin supplements.

THE WORKOUT

Now that you know how good exercise will make you look and feel, you are probably itching to do your first workout! FIRST, however, TURN BACK TO CHAPTER 1 AND DO YOUR WARM-UP EXERCISES – it is very important that you do not skip these.

Once you have warmed up, you will be ready to tone your muscles. REMEMBER TO FOLLOW THE POSTURE CHECK AND HEALTH AND SAFETY TIPS GIVEN IN CHAPTER 1 THROUGHOUT THE WORKOUT.

Repeat each exercise as many times as you feel able, starting with a moderate number of repetitions – say five – and increasing as you grow stronger. Do not overdo it the first time you exercise, you will only end up with sore muscles.

A note about abdominal exercises

Strong abdominal muscles will protect your back, as well as keep you looking trim, so it is well worth exercising them *before* you become pregnant in order to make your pregnancy easier, and to help you get back into shape more quickly afterwards.

Your abdominal muscles will be put under a lot of strain as your bump grows so NEVER over-exercise them when you are pregnant. The muscles have to stretch to accommodate your baby and sometimes will even separate, but usually they will return to normal after the birth. If you perform abdominal exercises which are too strong during pregnancy, the muscles may not close up again. So only perform the abdominal exercises given here BEFORE you become pregnant, NEVER once you are pregnant. When you have conceived, follow the appropriate workouts in Chapters 3, 4, 5 and 6.

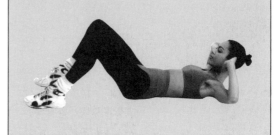

1 PELVIC TILT
You will have practised this already at the beginning of the warm-up, but good posture is essential to efficient exercise, so check your position again.

Stand with your legs apart and your knees directly over your ankles. Place one hand on your lower back and the other on your abdomen.

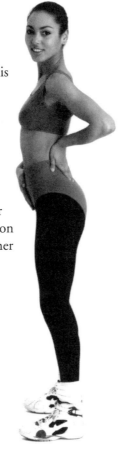

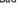

Bad

Tuck your hips and bottom under and forwards to tilt your pelvis. Come back to the centre and repeat. Make sure you keep the rest of your body still – just move your pelvis.

Good

2 PRESS-UPS
Kneel on all fours, with your arms a little wider than your shoulders and your hands facing ahead. Pull in your tummy muscles and tilt your pelvis forward. Make sure your back is straight.

Slowly bend your elbows and lower your upper body to the floor, keeping your back flat. Do not let it dip.

Gradually straighten your arms to lift your body up to the starting position. Do not lock your elbows straight. Repeat the whole sequence. The further your arms are from your knees, the more difficult the exercise will be.

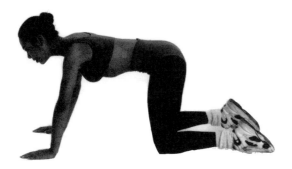

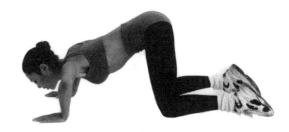

3 ABDOMINAL CURL-UPS

This is an excellent exercise for your abdominal muscles. Lie flat on the floor with your knees bent, tilting your pelvis and pressing the small of your back into the floor. Take your hands to the side of your head for support. Then, using your stomach muscles – not your hands – to lift you, carefully curl up, lifting your head and shoulders off the floor. Roll down gently again. Repeat. You should not allow your stomach muscles to bulge outwards as you do this. Breathe out as you come up and in as you go back down again.

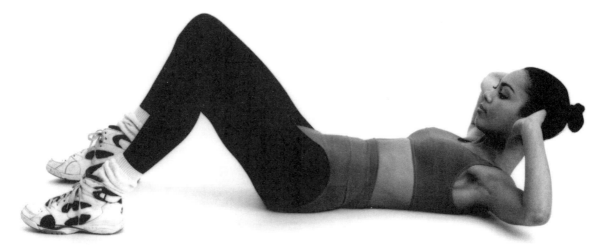

4 TO RELEASE YOUR STOMACH MUSCLES

Lie on your back with your knees bent, then roll your knees down to the floor on one side, while rolling your arms out to the other side. Repeat in the opposite direction. You should feel your muscles release.

5 PELVIC FLOOR

Before you become pregnant, you may find it easiest to exercise your pelvic floor while you are on your back with your knees bent and feet flat, so do some pelvic floor exercises now. See Chapter 1 if you need a refresher on how to do them.

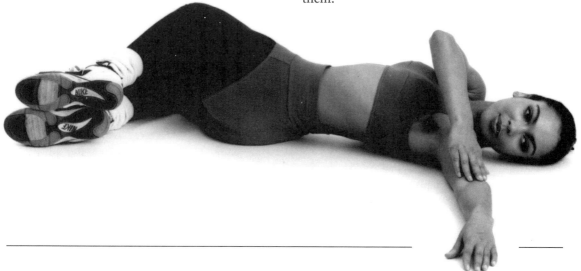

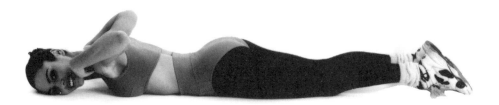

6 TRAPEZIUS PRESS

Lie on your tummy with your elbows bent at shoulder height and your hands on your shoulders. Keeping your head on the floor, turned to one side for comfort, raise your arms off the floor and draw your elbows up towards the centre of your back. You should feel your chest open out. Lower your arms again slowly. Repeat.

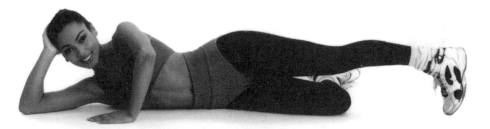

7 OUTER THIGH

Lie on your side in a straight line, with your bottom leg bent underneath for support. Rest your head on your hand and place your other hand in front of you on the floor. As you look down your body, your shoulders, hips and feet should all be in a straight line and facing ahead.

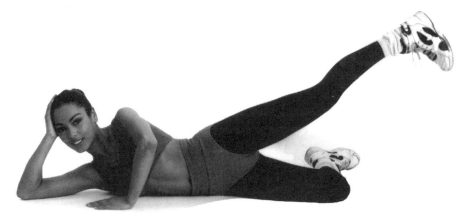

Pull in your tummy muscles and lift your upper leg slowly upwards towards the ceiling, making sure that you do not rock the rest of your body back. Keep the side of your leg facing upwards, the front of your thigh facing forwards. Then slowly lower the leg to just above the starting position and repeat. Allow your leg to come down to the floor.

8 INNER THIGH

In the same position, bend the top leg, so that your knee is bent and the leg is in front of you. Keep your lower leg straight and in line with your body.

Lift up the lower leg slowly, and then lower it again without letting it touch the floor. Repeat, then let your leg come down to the floor.

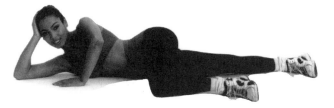

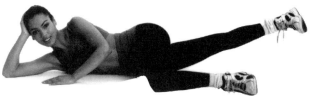

Now change sides and repeat exercises 7 and 8.

9 BUTTOCKS AND BACKS OF THIGHS: LEG RAISE

Lie on your tummy and lift one leg slowly up, then down in a straight line behind you, keeping your hips on the floor. Repeat. Now repeat with the other leg.

10 BUTTOCKS AND BACKS OF THIGHS: LEG CURL

In the same position, bring the lower half of one leg in towards your bottom by about 45°, and then slowly take it out again. Repeat, then repeat with the other leg.

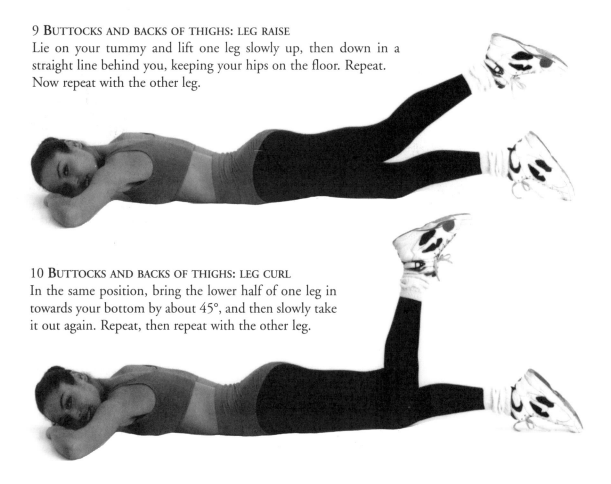

Cool down

Letting your body temperature revert to normal gradually is as important as the warm-up you do before exercise. These gentle stretches will reduce the chance of you feeling any stiffness or soreness after exercising. Hold each stretch for a count of six to eight. Do not stretch for longer than is comfortable.

12 TRICEP STRETCH

Still sitting, take your left arm behind your head, bending at the elbow. Use your right hand to gently ease the left elbow down behind your head. Then change arms to stretch the right tricep.

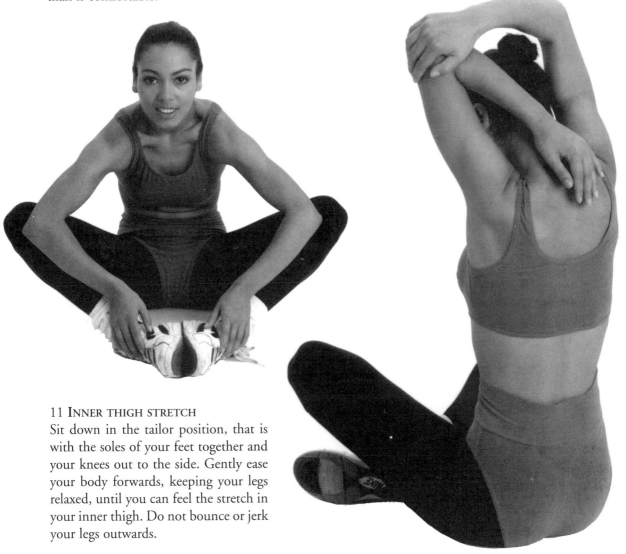

11 INNER THIGH STRETCH

Sit down in the tailor position, that is with the soles of your feet together and your knees out to the side. Gently ease your body forwards, keeping your legs relaxed, until you can feel the stretch in your inner thigh. Do not bounce or jerk your legs outwards.

13 PECTORAL STRETCH
Still sitting, take both arms right behind your back and clasp your hands loosely. Ease your arms straight back to push your chest open.

14 TRAPEZIUS STRETCH
Now take your arms in front of you and clasp your hands. Stretch forwards as far as you can, while keeping your back up straight. Feel the stretch across your upper back.

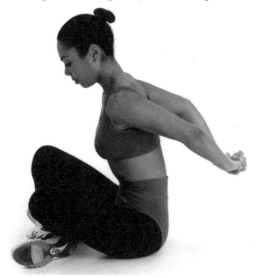

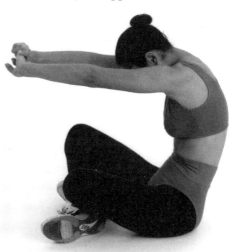

15 HAMSTRING STRETCH
Lie on your back with your left leg bent and the foot flat on the floor. Raise your right leg up towards the ceiling, hold it behind the thigh and bring the leg gently towards you, so you can feel the stretch along the thigh. Repeat with the other leg.

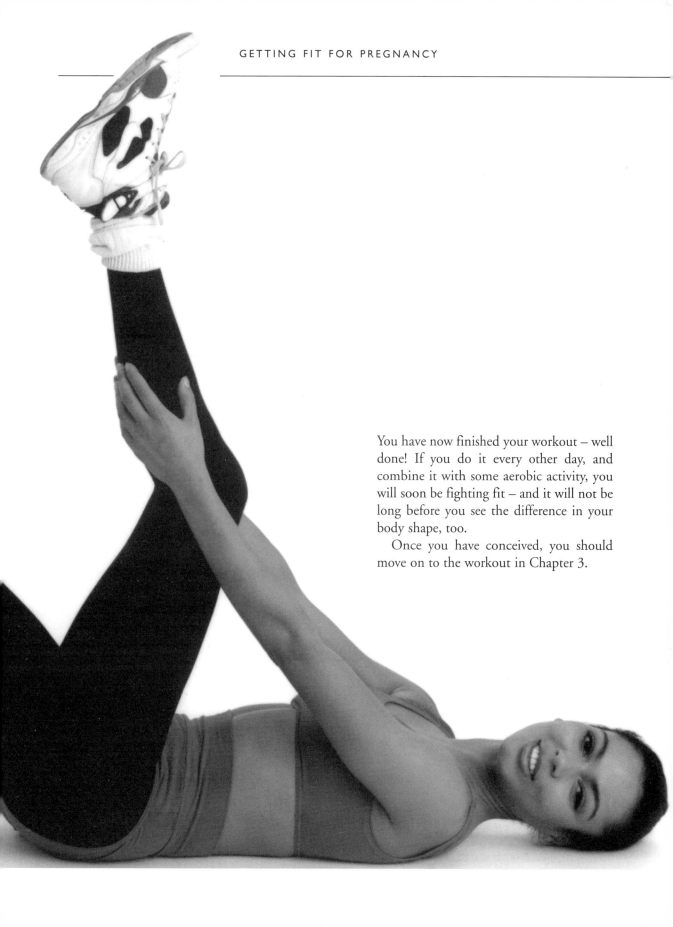

You have now finished your workout – well done! If you do it every other day, and combine it with some aerobic activity, you will soon be fighting fit – and it will not be long before you see the difference in your body shape, too.

Once you have conceived, you should move on to the workout in Chapter 3.

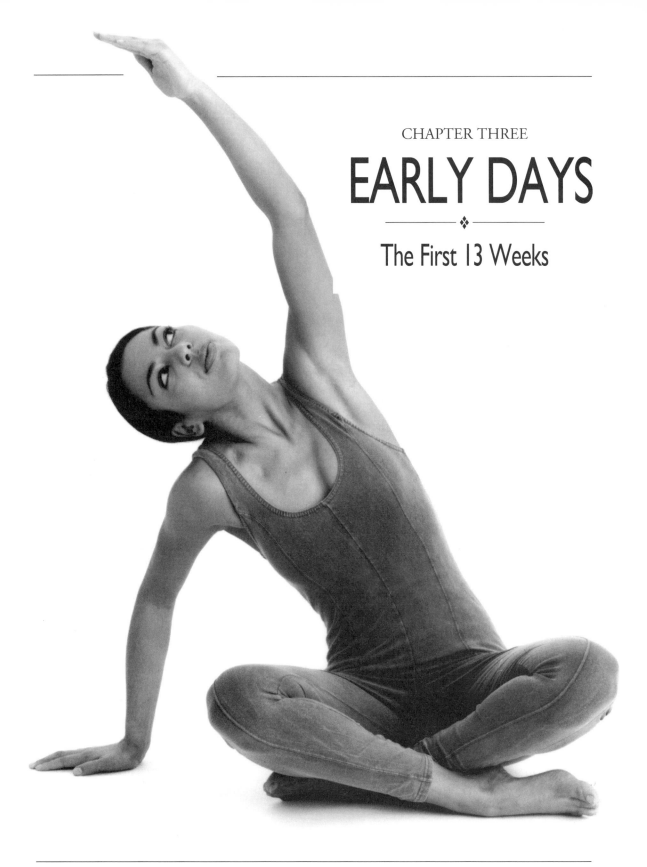

CHAPTER THREE

EARLY DAYS

❖

The First 13 Weeks

CONGRATULATIONS, you are pregnant! You are now embarking on the exciting journey to motherhood, and the fun starts here. You may be one of those women who feels 'different' as soon as they conceive, or you may find it strange that you feel no different at all, but either way, you can be sure that your body is now undergoing a lot of changes. The more aware you are of these changes, the more you will understand your body and know its limitations, both of which are vital to a fit, healthy pregnancy. It is important to get the right balance between getting enough exercise and overtaxing your body.

YOUR MUSCLES AND LIGAMENTS

The bones of your pelvis are held together by bands of fibrous, flexible tissue called ligaments. These are designed to prevent you moving your pelvis excessively or abnormally and will normally become taut when the pelvis reaches its limit of movement. Now that you are pregnant, however, the pregnancy hormones released by your body cause these ligaments, and other ligaments around your body, to swell and soften in preparation for the birth. This means that their 'safety mechanism' does not work so well, and you will have to be more careful when you exercise in order not to over-stretch them.

Additionally, as your baby gets larger and heavier, your pelvis is inclined to tilt forwards. This alters your posture and puts extra strain on the already soft ligaments and muscles in your lower back. This explains why you have to take so much more care of your back now that you are pregnant and why you must be careful when you are exercising, lifting and lowering heavy things and getting up and down from the floor (see pages 37–8).

HOW YOU WILL LOOK

Once you are pregnant, your breasts will become heavier than normal and the areola (the darker skin around the nipple) will appear to enlargen and become more bumpy as little nodules grow there in preparation for breast-feeding. You may notice blue veins becoming more prominent too, as the blood supply to your breasts increases.

Your waistline will probably not look very different until the end of this 'trimester' – about 12 weeks – but your uterus is already enlarging and its muscle fibres are thickening.

You may also find that your skin and hair change, for the worse or better, as the pregnancy hormones take effect.

HOW YOU WILL FEEL

Your growing uterus is pressing on your bladder, so you will probably be dashing to the lavatory rather frequently. Your breathing will become quicker too, so that you can send more oxygen to your growing baby.

You may also be suffering from the infamous morning sickness, which in fact can last all day, or simply occur in the evening instead. If you do feel nauseous, try eating several small meals a day instead of three large ones, and keep a supply of dry biscuits to hand to nibble on when nausea strikes.

It is likely that you will also feel extremely tired. After all, your body is doing a lot and it will take its toll. Do not fight fatigue: put your feet up and relax whenever you can.

If you are suffering from tiredness and sickness, exercising is sometimes the last thing you feel like doing. Do not worry: you will begin to feel better by about the 11th week, but in the meantime do try at least to do the gentle stretching exercises in the warm-up section (see

Chapter 1), even if you cannot face a whole workout. When you are feeling sick, a walk in the fresh air may help you feel better – so you can settle your stomach and exercise at the same time!

CAN I? CAN'T I?

Now you are pregnant, you will have to be a bit more careful about the sort of exercise you do – and you have taken the first important step by buying this book! Follow the guidelines given here and you and your baby will stay fit and well. If you have any doubts or worries about any exercise, speak to your doctor.

For the first trimester, you should be able to continue with most of the sports that you already do – as long as you feel well enough – but there are some activities you should avoid.

- **Sit-ups**   The muscles that run vertically down your stomach (the longitudinal muscles) are designed to separate as your baby grows. Once your baby is born they should return to their original state (with the help of the exercises shown later in this book), but if you over-stretch them while you are pregnant, it can slow down their recovery.

  Even sitting up straight from a lying-down position separates the longitudinal muscles, so you should never do any exercise that puts any strain on them, and follow the instructions on page 38 for how to get up and down from the floor.

- **Contact sports**   Any activity where you are likely to get hit, shoved or fall accidentally is not advisable once you are pregnant. Your baby is very well protected in your stomach, but it is still not worth the risk. You also do not want to risk injuring yourself at this important time.

- **Horse riding and skiing** Unless you are very proficient at these, it is advisable to stop doing both from the second trimester, when you are

getting larger, until after the baby is born. The extra weight in front of you changes your balance, and gives you less control.

- **Jogging** You may not find jogging very comfortable now anyway with your newly heavy breasts, but it should be avoided in any case, because of the damage the jarring action can inflict on your softened joints – especially your back, pelvis and knees.

Be careful

At the risk of being a complete killjoy, there are also some foods that you should avoid as soon as you become pregnant. Your baby does not yet have the same immune system as you, and so is much more vulnerable to infection. Cut out the following:

- **Soft cheeses** These include camembert and brie, goat's cheese, blue-veined cheese and sheep's milk cheese. These contain the listeria bacteria which can give you listeriosis. This will simply feel like a dose of 'flu to you, but to the developing baby it can be fatal. Also be careful of **cooked and chilled food**, as bacteria multiply in these conditions.

- **Raw eggs** Salmonella is always a risk with raw eggs and with chicken that has not been properly cooked. Be careful to cook both of these throughout your pregnancy and avoid any mayonnaise and mousse which contain raw eggs.

- **Liver and foods containing liver**   These contain a high level of vitamin A, which can harm a developing baby.

MIND AND SOUL

So much for the body. Your emotional fitness is, of course, just as important, and deserves equal attention, both now and after you have had the baby.

Hormones become a key word in pregnancy, and can become a good excuse for any problem you have, but you really cannot overestimate the effect that the flood of pregnancy hormones in your body has on how you feel. In the first three months especially, you may find that you swing from happiness to despair in a matter of minutes, or that you burst into tears at the smallest thing. Explain to your partner what is happening, and that you will get back to normal eventually. Hopefully, he will be patient and understanding.

Do not worry if you do not feel as happy and excited as you expected to be when you became pregnant. Firstly, you are having to cope with all the physical discomforts already mentioned, and that can leave you feeling slightly low. But even more frustrating can be all the doubts and concerns that insist on sneaking into your mind. Even women who have been trying for a baby for a long time can find it a bit of a shock when the dream becomes a reality. It is not surprising. What you are embarking on is a life-changing event, and if this is your first baby you are moving into unknown territory, so to feel unprepared and nervous is perfectly normal. Your partner probably feels the same way as well, so try talking to him about his feelings and helping one another through it.

Exciting and daunting as having a baby is, it is also important not to let it dominate your life now. You can be sure you will have little time for anything else once the baby has been born, so make the most of this 'free' time to enjoy life to the full. Meet your friends, go out, perhaps even go on holiday, and try not to talk 'baby' all the time – you will feel much better for it.

WORK MATTERS

There is no reason why you should not continue to work for as long as you feel fit and healthy, but it may be difficult from time to time. You may not want to tell everyone that you are pregnant until the 12th week, when the risk of miscarriage has lessened, so they are not going to understand why you are making frequent trips to the lavatory, eating strange things and bursting into tears at the slightest thing. It can make it easier if there is someone there that you can confide in. He or she can be a shoulder to cry on when the going gets tough.

Later in your pregnancy, you will be feeling tired and large, and may find that the stresses of work are taking their toll. Try to take it easy. Do not go rushing around in your lunch hour and ask if you can perhaps alter your hours slightly in order to avoid travelling in the rush hour. Remember that you and the baby are more important than your work or the latest deadline.

LOOKING AFTER YOUR BACK

Hormones soften your ligaments during pregnancy, and the sacroiliac joints of your lower back and the symphysis pubis (your front pubic bones) expand slightly to give your baby more room during labour. This makes your back more vulnerable than before and you should be careful how you lift, bend, sit down and get up.

Lifting

The golden rule here is to bend your knees, not your back. Let your thighs take the strain.

- Get close to whatever you wish to lift.
- Bend your knees and keep your back straight.
- Hold the object close in to your body.
- Use your leg muscles to raise yourself up again.
- Do not twist your body as you move.

To get down to the floor

A lot of the exercises in this book will require you to lie on the floor, so make sure that you know how to get up and down without putting your back at risk BEFORE you start the workouts.

1 Gently go down on to one knee, keeping your back as straight as possible. Then bring your other knee down.

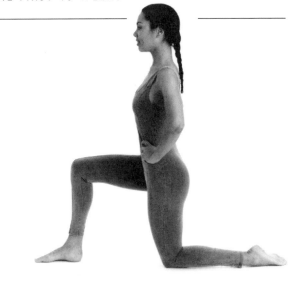

2 Take your hands to one side of you and rest them on the floor, so that they can support your weight as you shift your bottom to one side on the floor.

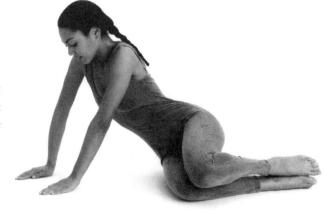

3 Ease your legs out to the side and lower your upper body slowly to the floor.

To get up from the floor

Reverse the sequence given above.
1 Lie on your side, up on your hip. Lift your upper body so that you are kneeling, and bring one leg up in front of you.

2 Put your hands on your upper thigh and use the muscles in your legs to help you up from the floor. Try not to push down on to your thigh.

THE WORKOUT

BEFORE YOU START YOUR WORKOUT, TURN BACK TO CHAPTER 1 AND DO YOUR WARM-UP EXER-CISES. REMEMBER TO FOLLOW THE POSTURE CHECK AND HEALTH AND SAFETY TIPS GIVEN IN CHAPTER 1 THROUGHOUT THE WORKOUT.

Now you are warmed up, you are ready to begin. Only do as many repetitions as are comfortable, and increase the number as you grow stronger.

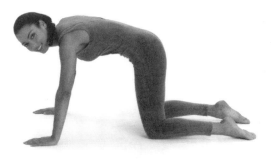

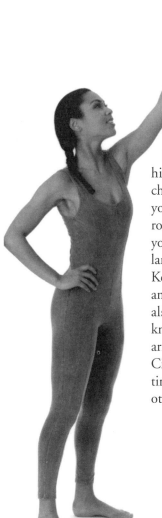

1 ARM CIRCLES

Stand with your feet hip-distance apart and check your posture. Circle your right arm up and round, keeping it close to your ear and drawing as large a circle as possible. Keep the movement slow and controlled. You could also try bending your knees as you circle your arms for more movement. Circle your right arm four times, then repeat with the other arm.

2 PRESS-UPS

Kneel on all fours, with your arms a little wider than your shoulders and your hands facing ahead. Pull in your tummy muscles and tilt your pelvis forward.

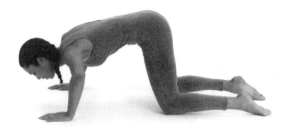

Slowly bend your elbows and lower your upper body to the floor, keeping your back straight – do not allow it to dip.

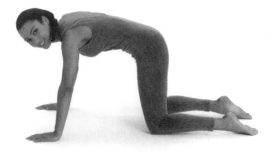

Gradually straighten your arms to lift your body up to the starting position. Do not lock your elbows straight. Repeat the whole sequence five times.

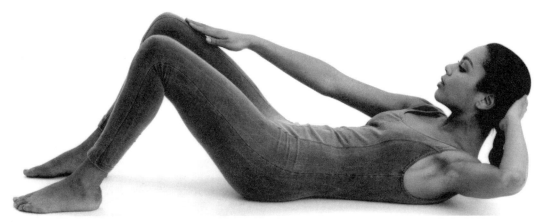

3 ABDOMINAL CURL-UPS

Lie flat on the floor with your knees bent, pressing the small of your back into the floor by tilting your pelvis. Put one hand at the side of your head for support and rest the other one on your thigh. Carefully curl up, using your tummy muscles, not your head, to lift your head and shoulders off the floor. Bring your resting hand up your thigh at the same time and keep your tummy muscles pulled in and flat. Roll down gently and repeat five times.

4 TO RELEASE YOUR STOMACH MUSCLES

Bend both knees into your chest and hold them there with your hands behind your thighs while your muscles relax. Then gently bring your knees back down again.

5 PELVIC FLOOR

You may still find it easiest to exercise your pelvic floor while you are on your back with your knees bent and feet flat. See Chapter 1 if you need a refresher on how to do the pelvic floor exercises.

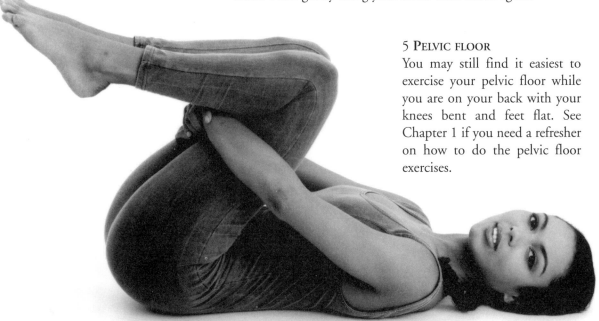

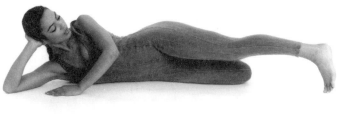

6 OUTER THIGH

Lie on your side in a straight line, with your bottom leg bent underneath for support. Rest your head on your hand and place your other hand in front of you on the floor. As you look down your body, your shoulders, hips and feet should all be in a straight line and facing ahead.

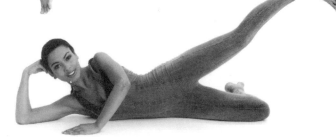

Pull in your tummy muscles and lift your upper leg slowly upwards towards the ceiling, making sure that you do not rock the rest of your body back and that the side of your top leg faces the ceiling. The front of the thigh should be facing forwards. Slowly lower the leg to just above the starting position and repeat ten times. Allow your leg to come down to the floor.

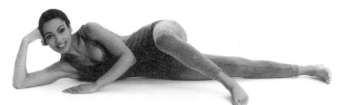

7 INNER THIGH

In the same position, bend the top leg and bring it in front of your lower leg, with the foot resting on the floor. Keep your lower leg extended straight along the floor in line with your body.

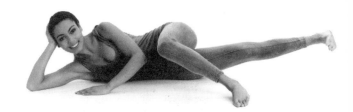

Lift up your lower leg slowly and then lower it again without letting it touch the floor. You will not be able to lift it very far, but you will feel it working the inside of your thigh. Repeat ten times, then let your leg come down to the floor.

Now repeat exercises 6 and 7 on the other side.

8 LEG RAISES

This exercises the buttocks and the backs of your thighs.

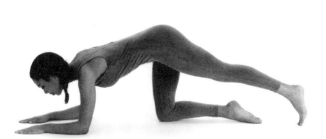
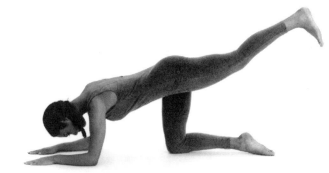

On all fours, lower yourself on to your elbows and tilt your pelvis. Keeping your back straight and tightening your tummy muscles, extend one leg out behind you.

Lift the extended leg slowly up and down in a straight line behind you for a count of ten. Take care not to let your back sag and keep your tummy muscles tightened.

9 LEG CURLS

This also exercises the buttocks and back of the thighs. In the same position as for the last exercise, extend one leg out behind you, in a straight line with your back as before. Now bring the lower half of your leg in towards your bottom by about 45° and then slowly take it out again. Again, it is important that you keep your tummy muscles tightened and your back straight, in order to protect it. Repeat ten times.

Change leg and repeat exercises 8 and 9.

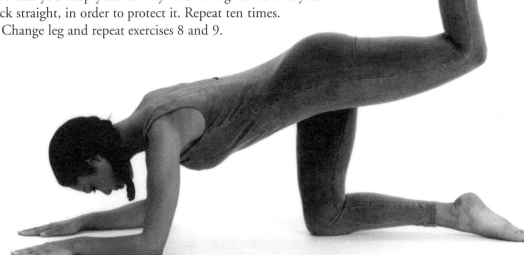

Cool down

These gentle, cooling-down stretches are especially important now that you are pregnant. Only hold each stretch for as long as is comfortable – a count of six to eight is ample.

1 QUADRICEP STRETCH
Lie on your tummy and bring one foot up behind you. Take hold of it with your hand and gently bring it up close towards your bottom without jerking. Hold it to feel the stretch at the front of your thigh, then release slowly and repeat with your other leg.

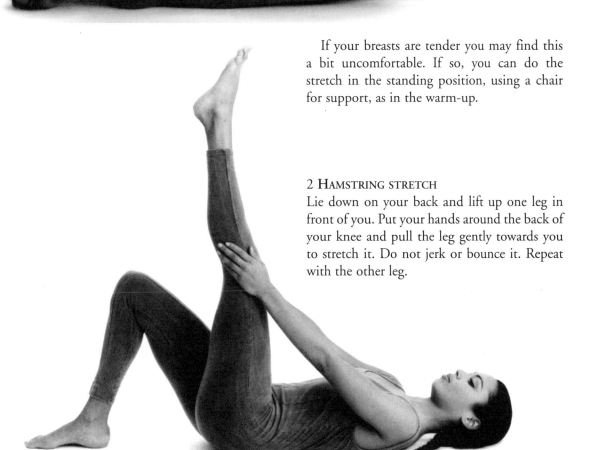

If your breasts are tender you may find this a bit uncomfortable. If so, you can do the stretch in the standing position, using a chair for support, as in the warm-up.

2 HAMSTRING STRETCH
Lie down on your back and lift up one leg in front of you. Put your hands around the back of your knee and pull the leg gently towards you to stretch it. Do not jerk or bounce it. Repeat with the other leg.

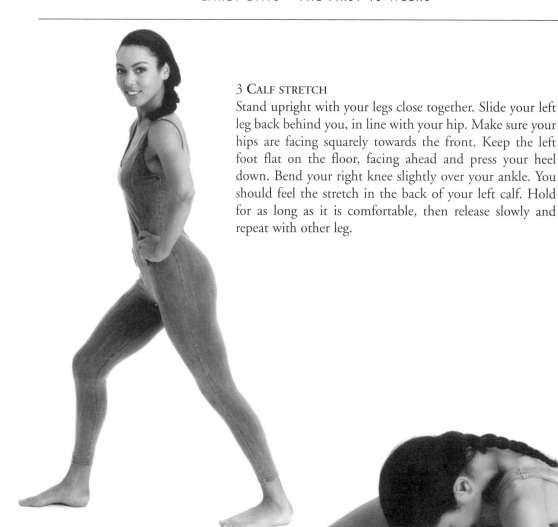

3 CALF STRETCH

Stand upright with your legs close together. Slide your left leg back behind you, in line with your hip. Make sure your hips are facing squarely towards the front. Keep the left foot flat on the floor, facing ahead and press your heel down. Bend your right knee slightly over your ankle. You should feel the stretch in the back of your left calf. Hold for as long as it is comfortable, then release slowly and repeat with other leg.

4 INNER THIGH STRETCH

Sit down with the soles of your feet together and your knees out to the side. Gently ease your body forwards, keeping your legs relaxed, until you can feel the stretch in your inner thigh. Do not bounce your legs down.

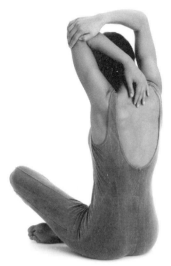

5 TRICEP STRETCH

In the same position, or cross-legged if you feel more comfortable, take your left arm behind the head, bending at the elbow. Use your right hand on the opposite elbow to gently ease the arm down behind your head. Feel the stretch in the arm. Then change arms to stretch the right tricep.

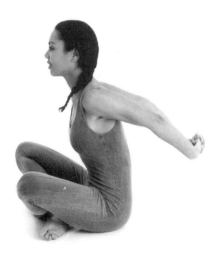

6 PECTORAL STRETCH

Still sitting in the same position, or cross-legged if you feel more comfortable, take both arms right behind your back and clasp your hands loosely. Push the arms gently straight behind you to open out your chest.

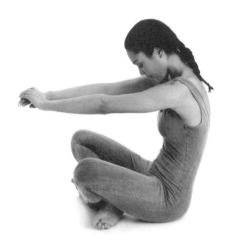

7 TRAPEZIUS STRETCH

Now take your arms in front of you, join your hands and stretch forwards as far as you can, while keeping your back straight.

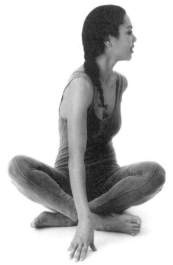

8 WAIST TWIST

Twist round at the waist to look behind you, keeping your hands on the floor. Be careful not to stretch too far, or strain your neck. Hold, then return to your starting position. Then turn to twist in the opposite direction.

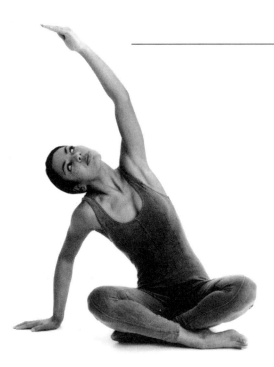

10 ARM STRETCH

Lift your left arm up above your head and stretch as far as you comfortably can. Slowly lower it and repeat with the other arm.

9 SIDE BENDS

Lift your left arm up and over your head and slowly bend over to the right, keeping the other arm on the floor for support. Feel the stretch down your left side. Hold it, then return to the centre and repeat to the other side.

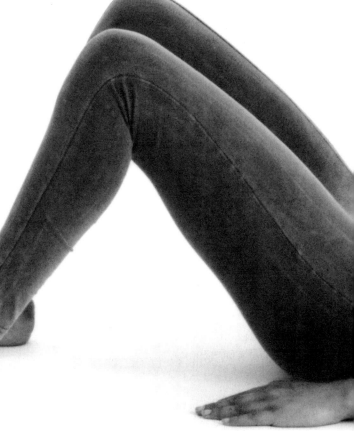

11 RELAXATION

Most of us lead such hectic lives that we rarely make time just to relax, but now that you are pregnant you need to listen to your body more and slow things down a bit from time to time, especially in the early and later stages of pregnancy. It may sound ridiculous, but it is often hard to let go completely. You need to relearn how to relax and feel how good it can be. Here's how:

- Take the phone off the hook and make yourself comfortable. You may want to play some relaxing music, or tape yourself reading these instructions as a reminder.

- Close your eyes and try to relax your body, so that you can feel it sink into the floor, bed or chair. Now slowly focus on every part of your body, starting at your toes and working up to your head, and concentrate on relaxing each one a little bit more.

- Soften your feet, calves, knees and thighs.

- Release your buttock muscles and try a pelvic tilt to prevent your back fron arching.

- Think about your fingers. Unclench them, stretch them out and let them curl back.

- Bring your shoulders down and concentrate on relaxing your neck area.

- Are you clenching your teeth? Open your mouth slightly, by dropping your bottom jaw, and let your tongue rest on the roof of your mouth. Moisten your lips.

- Imagine you are smoothing out any wrinkles on your face and forehead, and over your scalp.

Now you are completely relaxed, stay quiet and still for as long as you want to, listening to the gently rhythm of your breathing.

You have now finished your workout – well done.

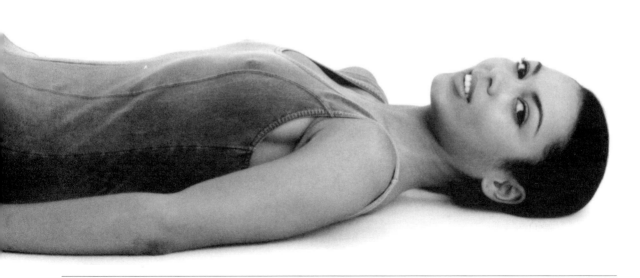

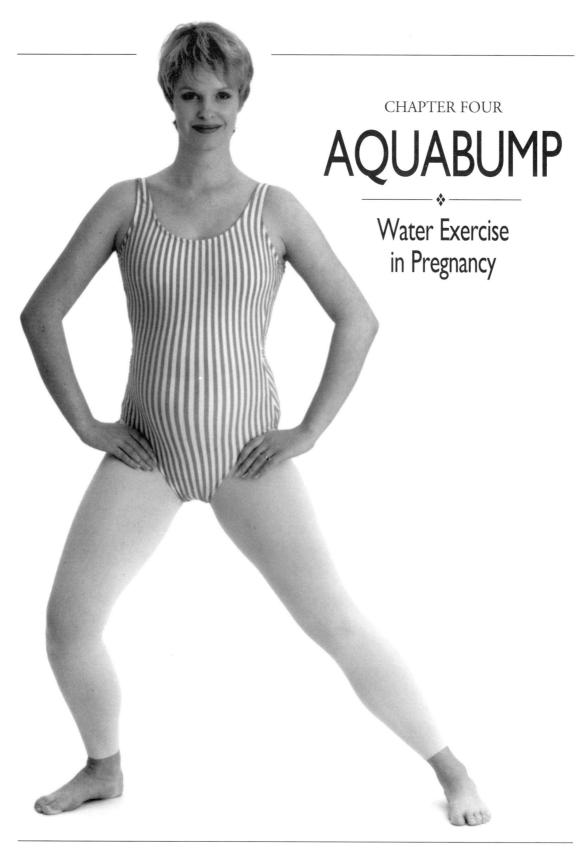

CHAPTER FOUR

AQUABUMP

❖

Water Exercise
in Pregnancy

IF YOU WANT to enjoy keeping fit, variety is the key. However good a particular workout is, you will soon get bored if you keep doing the same thing day after day. Hopefully, you are already combining the exercises in this book with some aerobic activity (see page 24), but if you are still making up your mind what else to do, why not take the plunge?

Swimming is probably the best exercise for pregnancy. It works the whole body without requiring you to pound, strain or twist. The water also supports your weight – which is a wonderful feeling when your bump is getting bigger!

Swimming strengthens you for pregnancy and labour by working the muscles that help you support the weight of your baby and which are put under strain during birth. Midwives and obstetricians are great advocates of swimming for this reason. They are convinced that increasing your muscle strength, and strengthening your heart and lungs, improves your chances of an easier labour, and swimming is the easiest and safest way of doing this.

Swimming is also one of the best exercises you can do if you find your breasts have become uncomfortably heavy as a result of your pregnancy. It is excellent for strengthening the pectorals – the chest muscles that support your breasts. And if aching legs are a problem, that is another reason to take to water: a swim or a walk is often the answer.

A regular swim will keep you feeling good too. Your baby is currently floating in his own little pool of amniotic fluid, so relaxing in water is the most natural way of unwinding. Tensions seem to drift away in the waves and, as after any form of exercise, the hormones released by your body will put you on a natural high. Your self esteem should also go up a few notches as you realize that your muscle tone is improving and you are not putting on so many extra pounds as your other pregnant friends.

MAKING A START

If you can swim, try to do so two, or preferably three, times a week, but start off moderately and listen to your body. If you feel that twice a week is ample, that is fine. Even getting to the pool once a week will make a difference. Space the swims evenly throughout the week though, so that your body can rest in between, and do not push yourself too hard.

If you cannot swim, turn to page 51, after reading the safety tips given below.

At the poolside

Always be careful when you are around the pool edge, as it is likely to be slippery. Before you get into the pool, sit at the side with your legs in the water. Relax and enjoy the sensation of the water on your skin. Extend your legs out into the water and flex and extend your toes. Circle your feet ten times to the left, then ten times to the right. Then gently kick your feet up and down as if you were using them to swim. This helps to get the circulation going in your body and will warm you up slightly before you begin to exercise.

Getting in

Use the steps or ladder to get into the water if you can. If not, sit on the side with your feet in the water and your hands on the pool edge by your sides. Press away from the side and slip gently into the water. Do not dive or jump in while you are pregnant.

WHICH STROKE?

Choose the stroke you feel happiest with, and the one you are most proficient at. If you do not breathe properly for the appropriate stroke you will run out of puff and get tired more quickly.

Crawl is recommended throughout pregnancy. It is easy to do, as the opposing arm and leg movements are similar to walking, although some people find the breathing more difficult to master.

Breaststroke is also recommended throughout pregnancy and is especially good for the third trimester, as it can be taken slowly and gently. You can also see better where you are going, and if anyone is in the way. As you become larger, you may find your feet break the surface of the water more often. Try dropping your knees down further before you extend your legs into a V-shape.

   If you have any back trouble it may be worth avoiding this stroke, as the inclination to try to keep your head out of the water encourages your back to over-arch.

Backstroke is a good stroke if you find breathing difficult with your face in the water – but you cannot see where you are going, so you will have to be more careful. It is good for toning your upper arms, which is helpful for the pushing stage of labour. Try using breaststroke leg movements as an alternative while you swim on your back, in order to exercise different muscles in your legs.

FROM BEGINNING TO END

You can continue swimming right up until the day you give birth if you wish, but consider the following points for each trimester:

First trimester Unless you are suffering from morning sickness or extreme tiredness, you should be able to swim as energetically as any non-pregnant woman. There is no need to modify your programme at this stage.

Second trimester As you begin to get a larger bump, you may find you have slightly less energy and you should be careful not to push yourself. Make your regular swim less demanding.

Third trimester You can still continue with regular gentle swimming, but avoid any strokes that feel uncomfortable and do not swim for so long. The breathing control that you need during swimming will be useful during child-birth, so concentrate on breathing in fully and deeply through your nose, and blowing out deeply through your mouth, as you do each stroke.

   If you prefer not to swim, simply do some of the stretching exercises given in this workout, or

---

Water, water everywhere!

A lot of pregnant women worry that if they swim or exercise in water too close to their due date they may not notice their waters breaking. There is a chance that you may not realize it has happened, but you will probably feel a warm gush of water. If this happens, leave the pool straightaway to reduce the risk of picking up an infection.

Dispelling the myths

• The chlorine in a pool will not cause you or you baby any harm. It is helping to keep the pool free of bacteria.

• You are unlikely to pick up a vaginal infection by swimming. Very little water actually enters the vagina while you swim.

---

float back in the water to relax. Now that your bump is larger, your specific gravity has changed too, and you will be even more buoyant!

STRETCH IT OUT

If you cannot swim, do not despair – you can still enjoy the benefits of exercising and relaxing in water while you are pregnant. Aquanatal classes, usually run by midwives, are springing up everywhere, so there is likely to be one at your local pool. If not, the routine given here will see you through your pregnancy.

THE AQUANATAL WORKOUT

This is the one workout in the book where you do not have to do the warm-up from Chapter 1 first. However, you can always incorporate parts of it into this routine if you wish.

Safety points

Although water is excellent at supporting you while you exercise, you should still be careful and listen to your body. Read the health and safety tips in Chapter 1 again and remember:

- Never swim alone.

- Do not swim when the pool is overcrowded – you do not want to be continually kicked or elbowed.

- If you experience any discomfort, slow down and take it easy.

- If you feel any pain – stop.

- Be very careful when you are walking around the pool – it may be slippery.

- Stop swimming if you feel too cold, too hot or too tired.

- Do not dive or jump into the water.

Repeat each exercise as many times as you feel able, aiming for just a few repetitions the first few times you do it and increasing as your muscles become stronger.

Warm-up

1 WATER WALK

Bob up and down in the water for 30 seconds, then walk slowly through the water for one minute: forward for eight paces, then back for four. Keep your arms relatively straight and push them forward and back at your sides as you walk so that the palms press against the water for extra resistance. This works the arms as well as the legs.

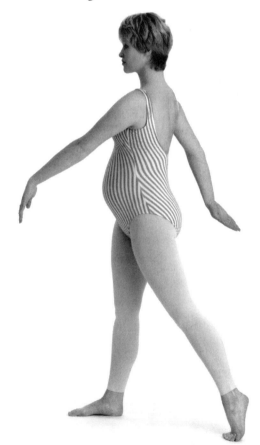

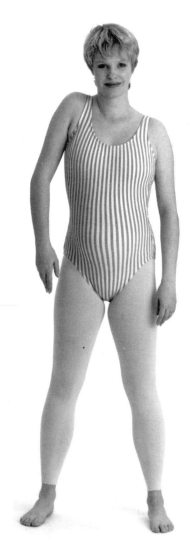
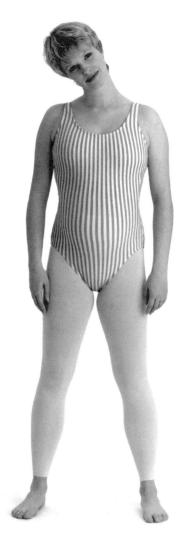
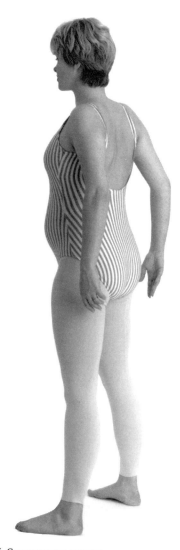

2 SHOULDER LIFTS
Standing waist-deep in water, check your posture, remember your pelvic tilt, and think tall. Lift your right shoulder up to your right ear without moving your neck or head, and then gently bring it back down. Repeat five times. Then repeat with the opposite shoulder.

3 NECK MOBILITY
Take your right ear towards your right shoulder, increasing the stretch gradually, and repeat. Repeat on other side. Try not to lift your shoulders as you take your ear down.

4 SHOULDER ROLLS
Roll your shoulders forward, and then press them down and backwards as if you were trying to get your shoulders to meet behind you. Repeat from the beginning.

Water workout

Now you are warmed up, you can start to work the different muscle groups. Remember to exercise your pelvic floor at some point during your workout too.

5 ARMWORK

Check your posture again, hold in your tummy muscles, remember your pelvic tilt and think tall. Lift your arms up at the sides, to shoulder level, keeping them straight *(right)*, then lower them again. Feel the resistance from the water and push against it as you come up and down. Keeping your hands stretched out and fingers closed together will increase the resistance and work your arms harder.

Increase the speed to make the arms really work.

Now continue the lift, to bring your arms above your head and down again.

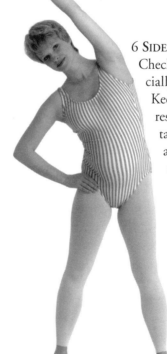

6 SIDE BENDS

Check your posture, especially your pelvic tilt. Keep your right hand resting on your hip and take your left arm up above your head and over to the right side. Be sure to keep your hips facing squarely forward and in one place. Repeat, then change to the other side.

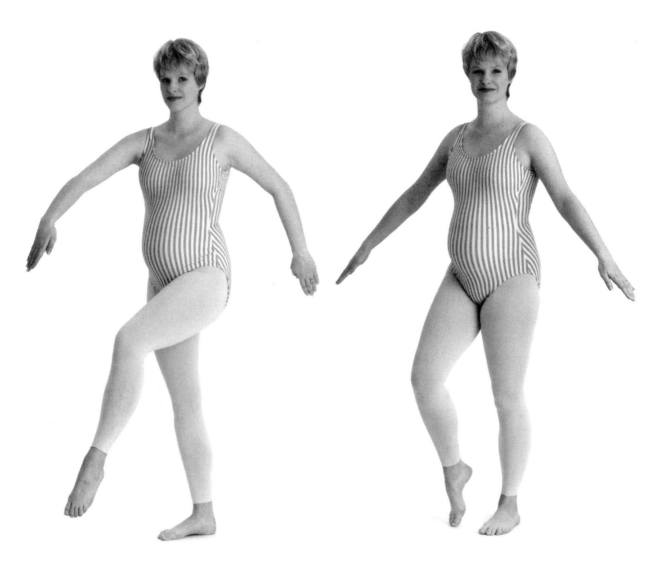

7 AQUAJOGGING
Stand in waist-deep water and jog slowly from one side of the pool to the other, moving your arms as if you were running and pushing against the water with them for extra resistance. Keep your fingers closed. Be careful to keep your balance. Repeat the lap if you wish. The water will give you extra support as you jog, but if you do not feel like jogging, you could walk instead.

8 ON-THE-SPOT JOGGING
Stand with your hands at your sides in waist-deep water, then jog in place, moving your hands in the water to keep you balanced and on the same spot. If you want extra bounce, push off the bottom of the pool.

9 PECTORALS

Stand in shoulder-deep water with your arms out at your sides, at shoulder height. Slowly bring your arms in together in front of you and then slowly out again, keeping your fingers closed in order to increase the resistance against the water. Do not move the rest of your body. Repeat.

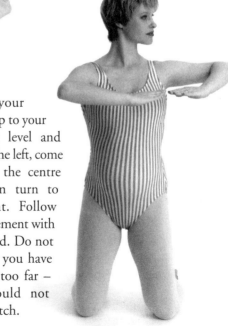

10 WAIST WORK

Go down on to your knees in the shallow end of the pool, pull in your bump and tuck your bottom under to check your posture, and move your knees hip-distance apart. Keep your back straight and tilt over to the side at the waist, reaching for the floor. Come back up to your starting point and repeat. Then repeat to the other side.

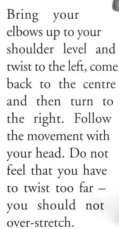

Bring your elbows up to your shoulder level and twist to the left, come back to the centre and then turn to the right. Follow the movement with your head. Do not feel that you have to twist too far – you should not over-stretch.

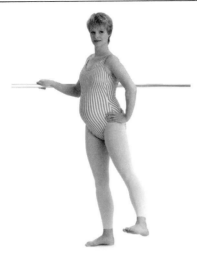

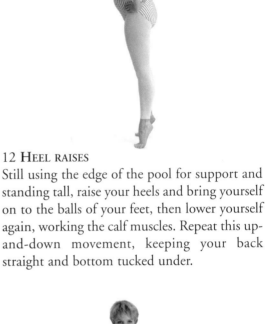

11 THIGH WORK

Standing in waist-deep water, check your posture. Pull in your abdominal muscles and tilt your pelvis. Holding on to the edge of the pool for support, take one leg out and up to the side, pushing your heel away from you against the water. Bring it in again and repeat. Turn to face the other way and repeat with the other leg.

12 HEEL RAISES

Still using the edge of the pool for support and standing tall, raise your heels and bring yourself on to the balls of your feet, then lower yourself again, working the calf muscles. Repeat this up-and-down movement, keeping your back straight and bottom tucked under.

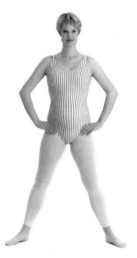

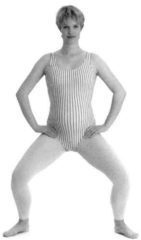

13 SQUATS

In shallow water, stand straight, with your legs slightly more than hip-distance apart and your hands resting on your hips.

Slowly lower yourself into a squat position – only as far as you can go while keeping your feet flat on the bottom of the pool and your knees apart. Keep your pelvis tilted and your bottom tucked under. Raise yourself carefully again and repeat.

Cool down

Holding these stretches for a count of six to eight should be sufficient. Never stretch for longer than is comfortable.

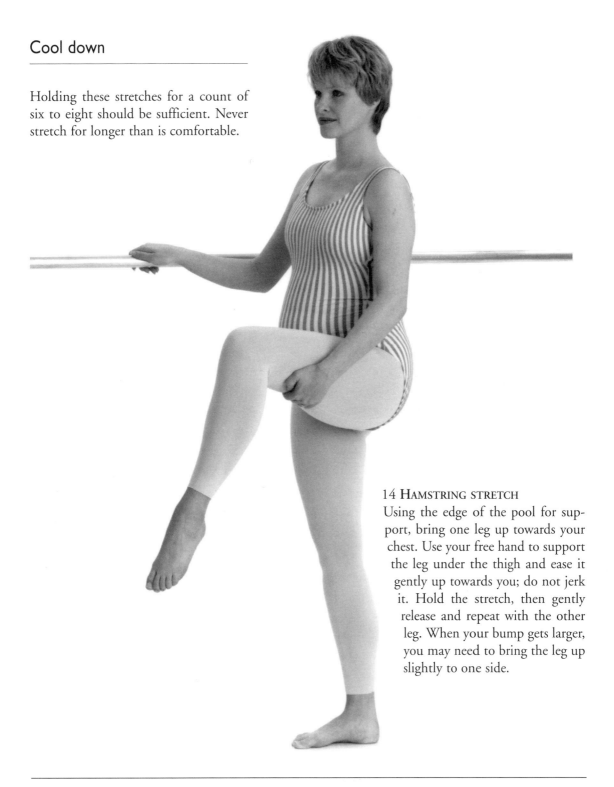

14 HAMSTRING STRETCH
Using the edge of the pool for support, bring one leg up towards your chest. Use your free hand to support the leg under the thigh and ease it gently up towards you; do not jerk it. Hold the stretch, then gently release and repeat with the other leg. When your bump gets larger, you may need to bring the leg up slightly to one side.

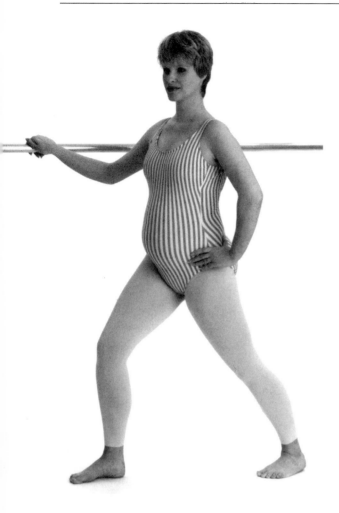

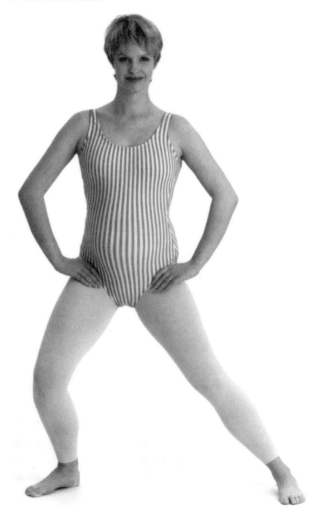

16 INNER THIGH STRETCH

Stand tall, with your hands on your hips and your legs slightly more than hip-distance apart. Bend your right knee out over your foot and, keeping your left leg straight, lunge slightly over your bent knee, until you feel the stretch in the inside of the thigh. Hold, then relax, come back to your starting position and repeat to the other side.

15 CALF STRETCH

Still holding on to the edge of the pool, take your right leg forward, and bend your knee out over your right foot. Keep your left leg straight behind you. Press your heel down on to the bottom of the pool to feel the stretch in the calf. Hold, then repeat with the other leg.

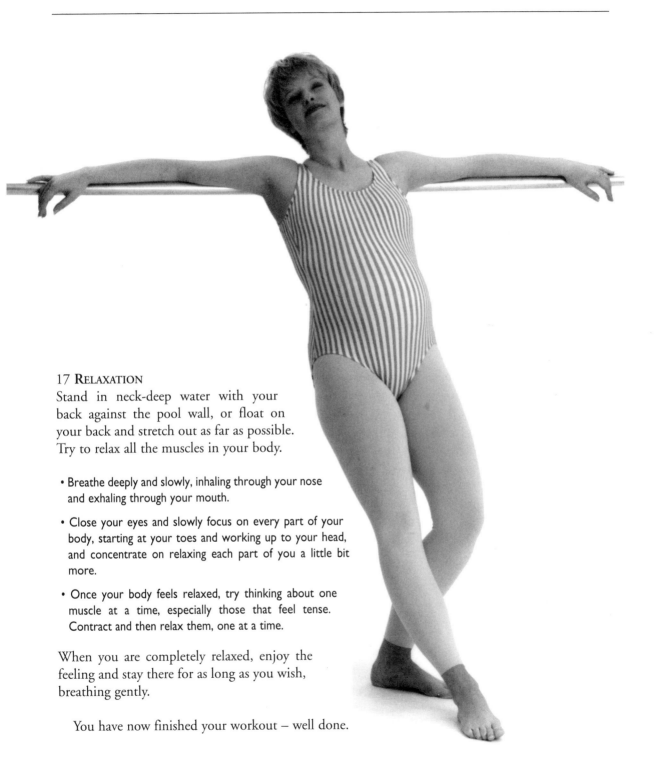

17 RELAXATION

Stand in neck-deep water with your back against the pool wall, or float on your back and stretch out as far as possible. Try to relax all the muscles in your body.

- Breathe deeply and slowly, inhaling through your nose and exhaling through your mouth.

- Close your eyes and slowly focus on every part of your body, starting at your toes and working up to your head, and concentrate on relaxing each part of you a little bit more.

- Once your body feels relaxed, try thinking about one muscle at a time, especially those that feel tense. Contract and then relax them, one at a time.

When you are completely relaxed, enjoy the feeling and stay there for as long as you wish, breathing gently.

You have now finished your workout – well done.

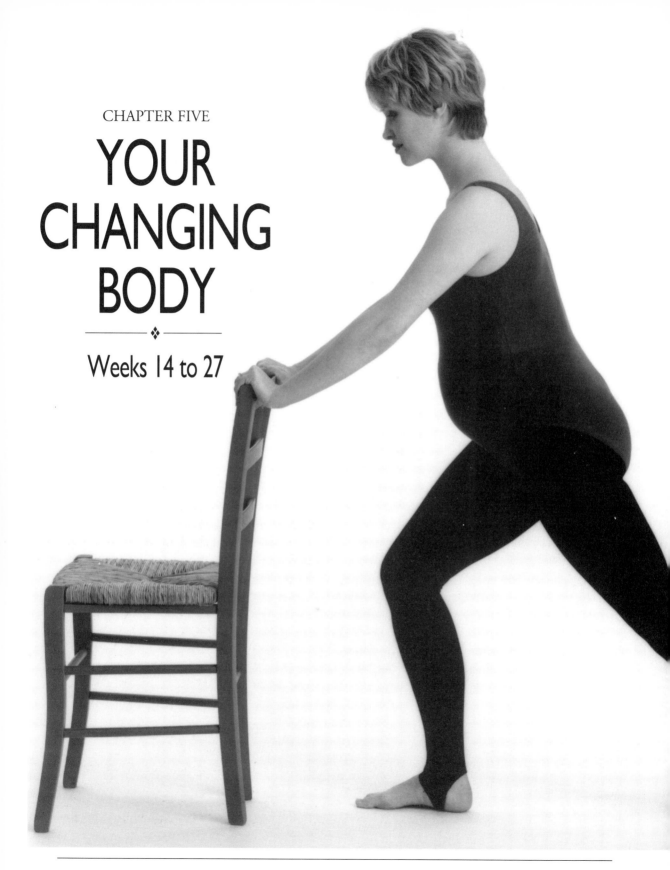

CHAPTER FIVE

YOUR CHANGING BODY

❖

Weeks 14 to 27

THE SECOND TRIMESTER is the period from 14 weeks to 27 weeks. Your baby is growing at an incredible rate and, by week 24, is likely to measure about 33cm (13in) long and weigh over 450g (1lb).

LOOKING GOOD

This is the time when a lot of women find that they feel better than ever before – positively blooming, in fact. Your bump is beginning to make itself seen, so you can prove to the world that you really are pregnant – not just plump! Morning sickness also eases by about the 11th week, and the pregnancy hormones released in your body often have the effect of making your hair shiny and your skin glow.

On the other hand, you may be one of the unlucky ones, and find that the same pregnancy hormones cause havoc with your body, making your hair unmanageable and your skin dry and patchy. If this happens to you, avoid putting anything dehydrating on your face (and that includes soap and water), use oils in your bath and try a milder shampoo. You may even want to consider having a shorter or easier to manage hairstyle while you are pregnant.

A HEALTHY BITE

Make sure you go to see your dentist now, and regularly throughout your pregnancy. The increased blood supply in your body and the hormone progesterone makes you more liable to gum problems, and you may find that they bleed when you brush your teeth. Visiting the dentist will ensure that you keep on top of any infections, but tell him that you are pregnant and do not have any X-rays. You are entitled to free dental treatment from the time you conceive to one year after your baby has been born, so make the most of it.

ACHES AND PAINS

Continuing with your exercise routine will keep you feeling on top form and help to prevent a lot of the common pregnancy niggles, but you may still find you suffer from a few aches and pains. Here are the most common complaints, and tips on beating them.

Backache Pregnancy hormones cause the ligaments of your spine to relax, so your hips and lower back are put under more strain than usual, especially with the extra weight of your growing baby. Stand up straight and check your posture in the mirror, using the photographs on page 63 as a guide. Maintaining good posture protects your back, and you should be particularly careful when you exercise. Avoid standing for long periods of time and wearing high heels.

Heartburn This is caused by stomach acid coming up into your oesophagus, creating a burning sensation. You may find it happens most when you are straining or lying down. Try eating smaller meals so that your stomach never becomes overfull, have a milky drink before bedtime to neutralize the acid and sleep propped up on pillows.

Cramp No-one seems to know for sure what causes cramp in pregnancy, but it could be due to salt deficiency or low calcium levels. Ask your partner to massage the area firmly, flexing your foot back up towards you whenever cramp strikes.

Feeling faint Your body is working very hard to develop your baby, and your uterus needs a lot more blood than usual, so you may feel light-headed now and then. When this happens, sit down with your head between your knees, or lie with your feet higher than your head until you feel better. Avoid standing for too long, or getting out of a hot bath too quickly.

Piles (haemorrhoids) As your baby presses on your rectum, it hinders the blood flow and encourages piles to develop. Keep eating plenty of fibre while you are pregnant to prevent piles developing, and avoid straining when you empty your bowels. Coughing and lifting weights also put a strain on your rectal veins, so avoid doing these if possible.

TOO SEXY?

Being pregnant is an exciting time for you as a couple, and a time when you can get really close – mentally and physically. However, it can be quite depressing to be told by books and experts how sexy you will feel at this stage, when in reality you would rather have a good night's sleep! Pregnancy affects everyone differently – some women just cannot believe how rampant they are (and their partners don't know what has hit them!), whereas others feel so sick, tired or aching that their libido hits an all-time low.

However you feel at the moment, do not worry: just go with the flow. It is likely that your libido will come and go as the pregnancy progresses, and you may feel quite different in another couple of months.

Your libido – or lack of it – has a lot to do with your self image too. If you see your growing belly and breasts as a wonderful expression of your femininity, or you are simply enjoying having a cleavage for the very first time, it is likely that you will want to share your lovely new body with your partner too. If, however, you believe your pregnancy has made you look fat or unattractive, it will stop you from relaxing and enjoying your body. Be confident about your changing shape. You are performing an

incredible feat, and your body is beautiful proof. The exercises and advice in this book will keep you shapely, supple and strong, so why not let you partner see how wonderful you are, too?

Providing you feel fine, you can continue to have sex with your partner right up until your baby is born, unless a professional has advised you otherwise for a medical reason. Sometimes, though, continuing your sex life is easier said than done. A growing bump can present new challenges. The classic man-on-top position will soon have to be abandoned, but you could try 'spoons', where you both lie on your side. A lot of pregnant women find they prefer to go on top, because they can then control the degree of penetration, and keep their breasts and bump out of the way.

Of course, there are plenty of other ways of staying close and intimate with your partner, even if you do not feel up to sex. Holding, touching and cuddling one another is just as good a way of communicating. Or why not try giving one another a sensual massage at the end of the day?

LEAVE MY BUMP ALONE!

Now that you really are beginning to 'show', you may find that your body – and even your life – is not your own. Deciding to have a baby is an important and personal decision for you and your partner, but you will probably find that your pregnancy is far from personal. As soon as you announce the good news, complete strangers will feel they have the right to comment on – and even prod at – your tummy. Conflicting or unwanted advice is likely to come flying from every corner, too: so much so, that you may just wish you could return to your old self now and then.

Whenever this happens, take a deep breath, and remember that it is your body and *your* baby, and ultimately, whatever anyone else says, how you look after them both is completely up to you. Everyone has their own ideas on pregnancy and babies, and a lot of them do conflict, so try to select one or two people whose views you respect, and turn to them alone for help if and when you feel you need it.

LOOKING THE PART

The time has come to wave goodbye to your jeans and skirts, and face the fact that your expanding waistline needs something a little more comfortable. Do not panic, you will not need to bid farewell to your fashion sense completely. Many high street stores stock decent maternity wear for the women who do not want to dress in pastel-coloured scout tents for the next few months. Many women find that a pair of leggings and some loose tops are all they need, but if you need to look smart for work, then you may have to buy a couple of dresses too.

It is important that you do not feel restricted and uncomfortable, especially when you are exercising. You do not have to wear the latest designer exercise gear: leggings and a cotton T-shirt will do. A well-fitting bra is a must, however. You will probably have gone up a size or two since you became pregnant, so go to a shop where they have trained bra fitters and check that you are wearing the right size.

Fancy footwork

Your feet may not have changed in size, but you should still give your footwear some consideration. High heels encourage bad posture and put an extra strain on your back, so go for shoes with no more than a 5cm (2in) heel. Look for designs which offer good support and preferably have a non-slip sole. Some women find

their feet do swell when they are pregnant, so you might need a half-size larger than normal. Trainers are ideal, and will come in useful if you are walking more to keep fit during your pregnancy. You do not have to wear trainers to do the exercises in this book, but if not, go bare foot instead – NEVER exercise in your socks or tights, as you could easily fall.

THE WORKOUT

BEFORE YOU START YOUR WORKOUT, IT IS IMPORTANT TO CHECK YOUR POSTURE. Now that your bump is beginning to show, it can be even more tempting to stick your stomach out and show it to the world. However, this makes your back arch and puts extra strain on it, which could lead to lasting back troubles. Instead, re-read the section on posture in Chapter 1 and check your position in a mirror. Notice the difference here between bad posture and good posture (see below). Not only will your body feel better as a result, you will also look slimmer and fitter.

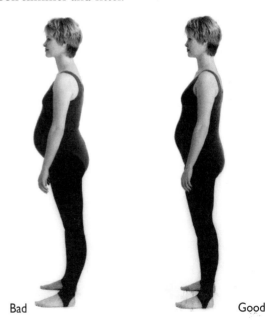

Bad   Good

NEXT, TURN TO CHAPTER 1 FOR THE WARM-UP SECTION or listen to your tape, if you have recorded the exercises, but take note of the following points:

- Omit the hamstring stretch on your back. You can do the same exercise standing up.

- Take care when you do the hip circles that you do not arch your back.

- Maintain your pelvic tilt and hold in your tummy muscles to give your back extra protection.

You are now ready to start the workout. The more you times you can repeat these exercises correctly, the more you will work the muscle groups, but do not strain yourself.

Aim perhaps to repeat each exercise five times at first, and build up to a level with which you feel comfortable.

1 CHEST OPENER
Stand with your feet hip-width apart, with your pelvis tilted and your tummy muscles pulled in. Think straight and tall, then round your back and bring both arms forward and slightly curved in front of you.

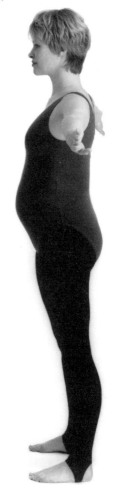

Open your arms out to the sides again, lifting and opening up your chest, but taking care not to arch your back as you do so. Breathe out deeply as you open out your arms.

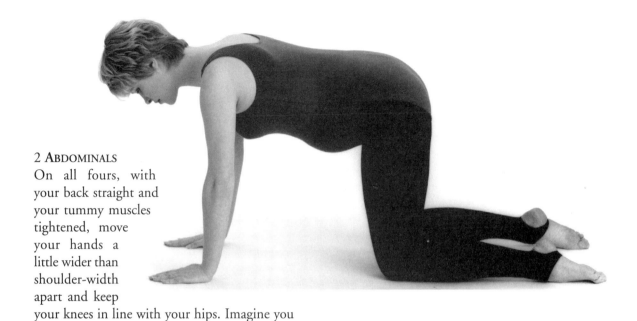

2 ABDOMINALS
On all fours, with
your back straight and
your tummy muscles
tightened, move
your hands a
little wider than
shoulder-width
apart and keep
your knees in line with your hips. Imagine you
are drawing a straight line from your bottom,
along your back and neck. Do not look
upwards.

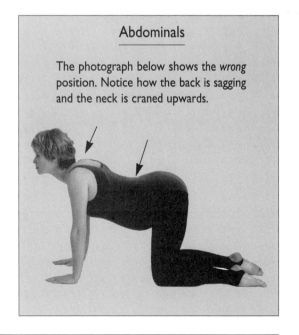

Abdominals

The photograph below shows the *wrong*
position. Notice how the back is sagging
and the neck is craned upwards.

Breathe out slowly, and at the same time, gently pull in your abdominal muscles and curve
your back upwards.

Return slowly to the start position and repeat.
Try not to lock your elbows. Stop immediately
if you feel at all sick or giddy.

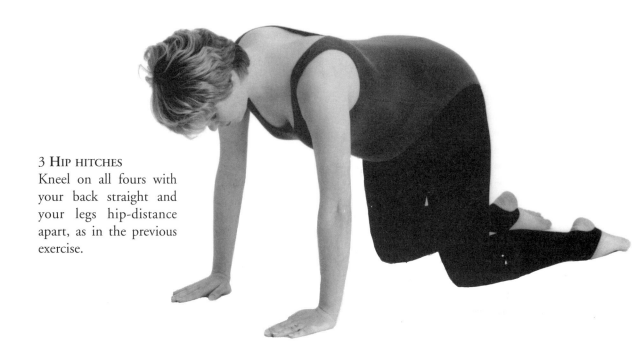

3 HIP HITCHES
Kneel on all fours with your back straight and your legs hip-distance apart, as in the previous exercise.

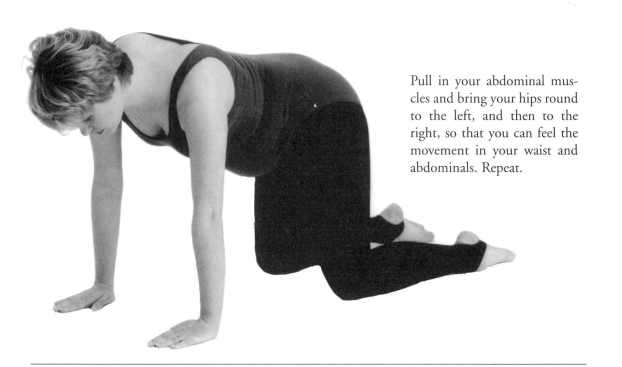

Pull in your abdominal muscles and bring your hips round to the left, and then to the right, so that you can feel the movement in your waist and abdominals. Repeat.

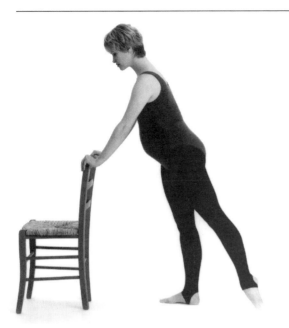

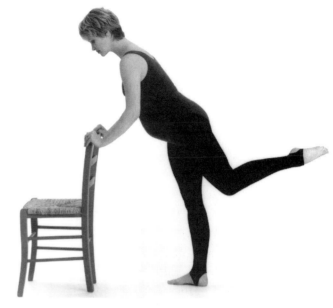

4 LEG CURLS

This exercises the buttocks and the backs of your thighs. Stand holding on to a chair or the wall for extra support, either facing it or sideways on. Maintain a pelvic tilt. Keep your feet flat on the floor and your knees slightly apart and bent. Pull in your tummy muscles and extend your right leg behind you.

Raise the leg a little way off the floor and hold it there. Bend the knee and bring the heel up towards your bottom, then lower it again slowly. Repeat. You will feel the back of your thigh working. Change legs and repeat the sequence.

5 LEG RAISES

This also exercises the buttocks and the backs of your thighs. Repeat the first part of exercise 4; then, keeping the right leg extended straight behind you, lift it up slowly, keeping it straight. You will not be able to bring it up very far. Make sure you keep your pelvis tilted forwards and do not arch your back. Lower it again and repeat as many times as you can before changing to the other leg.

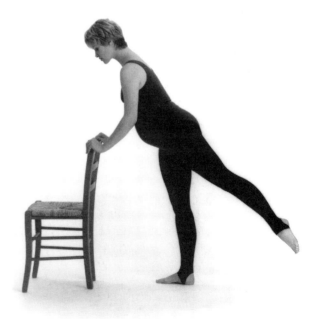

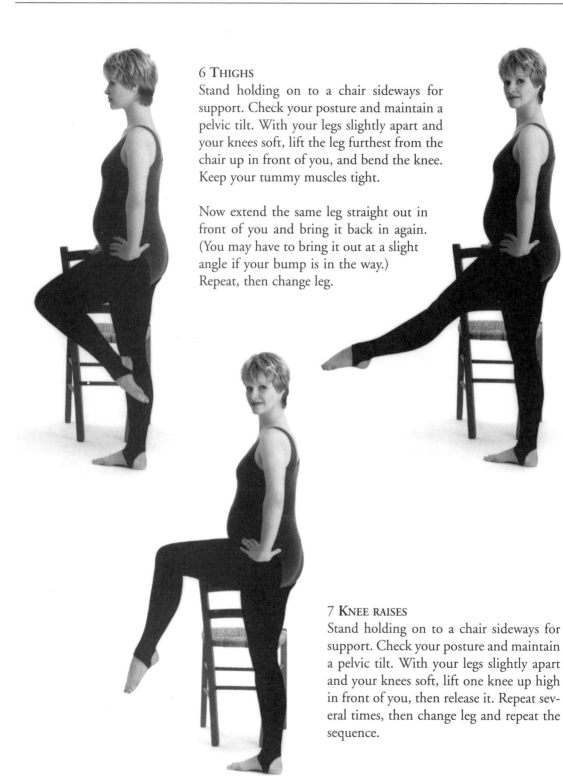

6 THIGHS
Stand holding on to a chair sideways for support. Check your posture and maintain a pelvic tilt. With your legs slightly apart and your knees soft, lift the leg furthest from the chair up in front of you, and bend the knee. Keep your tummy muscles tight.

Now extend the same leg straight out in front of you and bring it back in again. (You may have to bring it out at a slight angle if your bump is in the way.) Repeat, then change leg.

7 KNEE RAISES
Stand holding on to a chair sideways for support. Check your posture and maintain a pelvic tilt. With your legs slightly apart and your knees soft, lift one knee up high in front of you, then release it. Repeat several times, then change leg and repeat the sequence.

8 CHEST OPENER

This strengthens your upper body and can be done either standing or kneeling up. Put your hands on your shoulders, with your elbows raised up to shoulder height. Slowly draw your shoulder blades together behind you, keeping your elbows up. Release your shoulder blades and return to the centre. Repeat five times, taking care not to arch your back.

9 PRESS-UPS

Kneel on all fours, as in exercise 2, with your arms a little wider than your shoulders and your hands facing ahead. Pull in your tummy muscles and tilt your pelvis forward, making sure you keep your back straight. Then slowly bend your elbows and lower your upper body to the floor, keeping your back flat.

Gradually straighten your arms to lift your body up to the starting position, but do not lock your elbows straight. Repeat.

Cool down

Hold these stretches as long as you feel is comfortable; a count of six to eight should be sufficient. Do not push or bounce yourself into position.

10 CALF STRETCH
Hold on to the back of a chair with your hips facing squarely to the front. Check your posture.

Take one leg slightly behind the other. Bend the front knee over the ankle and keep the back leg straight, pressing your heel down into the floor. Hold to feel the stretch in your calf, then release and repeat the sequence with the other leg.

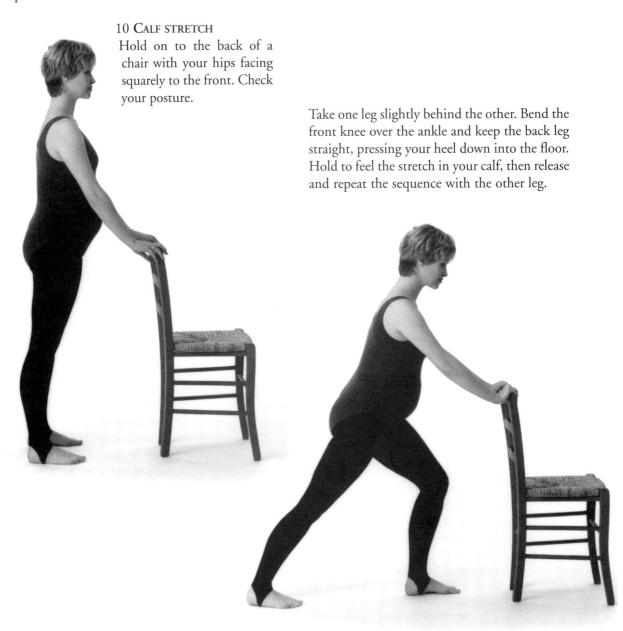

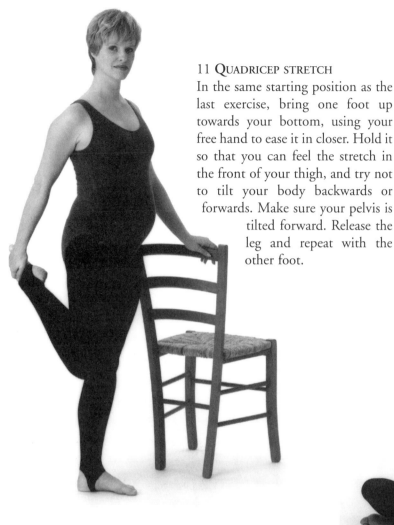

11 QUADRICEP STRETCH
In the same starting position as the last exercise, bring one foot up towards your bottom, using your free hand to ease it in closer. Hold it so that you can feel the stretch in the front of your thigh, and try not to tilt your body backwards or forwards. Make sure your pelvis is tilted forward. Release the leg and repeat with the other foot.

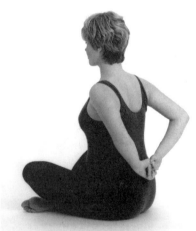

12 PECTORAL STRETCH
Carefully sit down in the tailor position (see page 31) or cross-legged and clasp your hands loosely behind your lower back, with your palms facing upwards. Bring your shoulder blades down, back and together, so that your elbows come closer and you can feel the stretch across your chest. Make sure that your lower back does not arch as you do it.

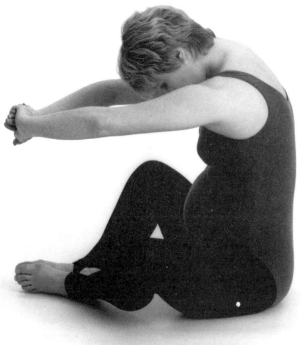

13 TRAPEZIUS STRETCH

Now stretch your arms out in front of you, clasp your hands loosely and round your back. Push your arms gently away from you to feel the stretch in the upper back.

14 TRICEP STRETCH

Circle both shoulders backwards a couple of times, then slowly lift one arm up above your head. Bend it at the elbow so that the lower half of your arm falls to your neck. Rest it there and gently use the other hand to ease the arm down your back as you stretch. Hold it, then gently release and change sides.

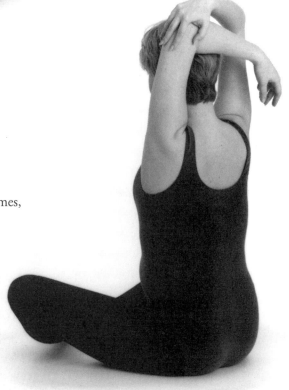

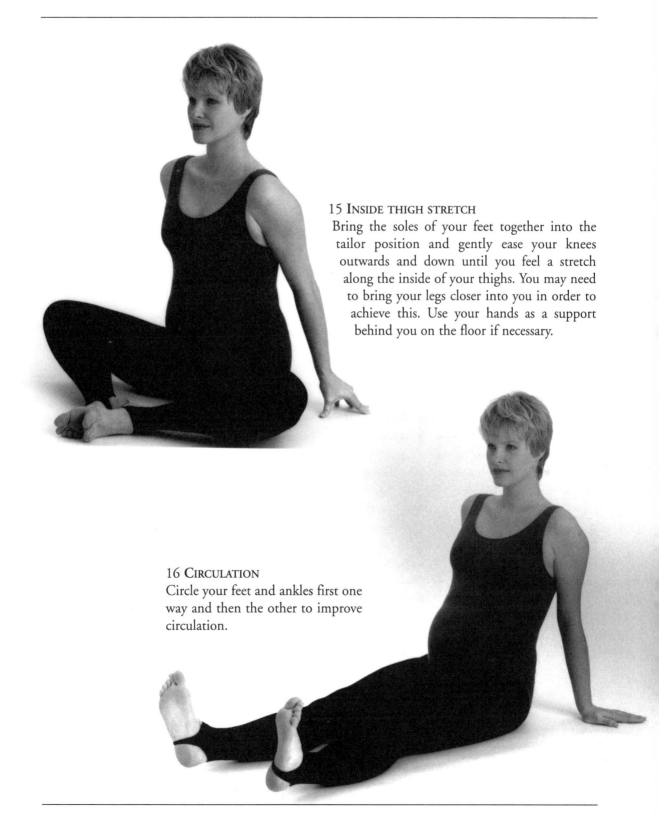

15 INSIDE THIGH STRETCH

Bring the soles of your feet together into the tailor position and gently ease your knees outwards and down until you feel a stretch along the inside of your thighs. You may need to bring your legs closer into you in order to achieve this. Use your hands as a support behind you on the floor if necessary.

16 CIRCULATION

Circle your feet and ankles first one way and then the other to improve circulation.

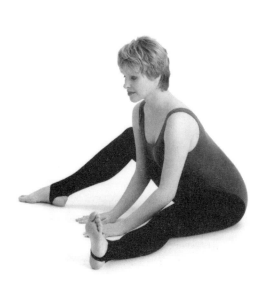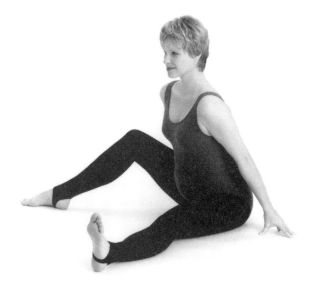

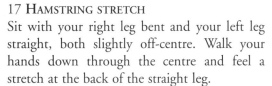

17 HAMSTRING STRETCH
Sit with your right leg bent and your left leg straight, both slightly off-centre. Walk your hands down through the centre and feel a stretch at the back of the straight leg.

Alternatively, place your hands on the floor behind you for support and gently ease your body forward. Hold to feel the stretch in the back of the leg. Change legs and repeat.

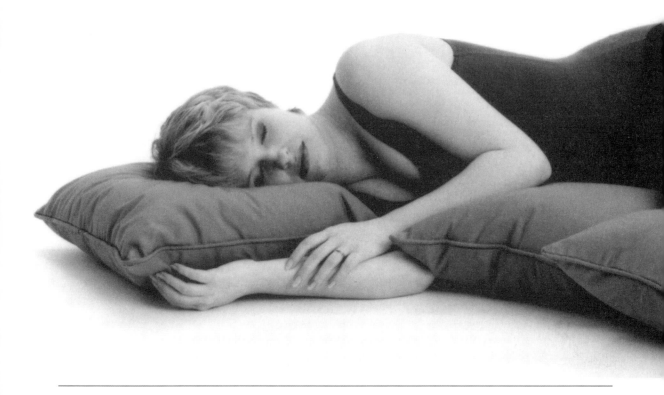

18 PELVIC FLOOR

Move carefully on to all fours and practise a few pelvic floor exercises.

RELAXATION

Now take some time out to unwind and relax. You may be feeling better than ever before at this stage in your pregancy, but you should not be tempted to push yourself at any time. Relaxation is still important.

- You should not be lying on your back now – you will probably find it too uncomfortable anyway. The baby is getting bigger and when you lie down will press on your large blood vessels, slowing your circulation. This will make you feel sick or dizzy, and may even be stopping the flow of oxygen to the baby.

- In order to help you get more comfortable on your side, use plenty of cushions or pillows. A cushion under your head, one under your bottom arm, one under your upper knee and perhaps even one under your bump will give you plenty of support. You may find this helps you sleep better in bed at night, too.

- Now that you are comfy, follow the same routine as in the last trimester. Lie back, close your eyes and take as long as you like to unwind completely.

You have now finished your workout – well done.

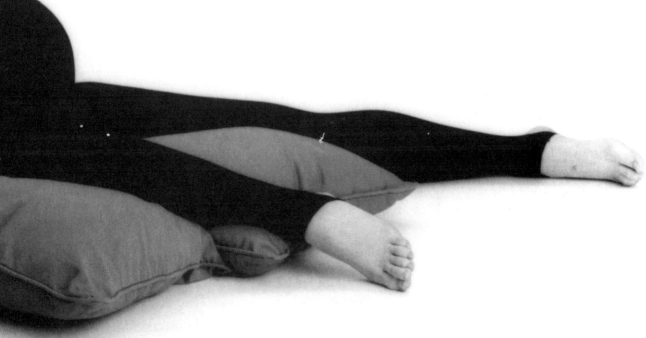

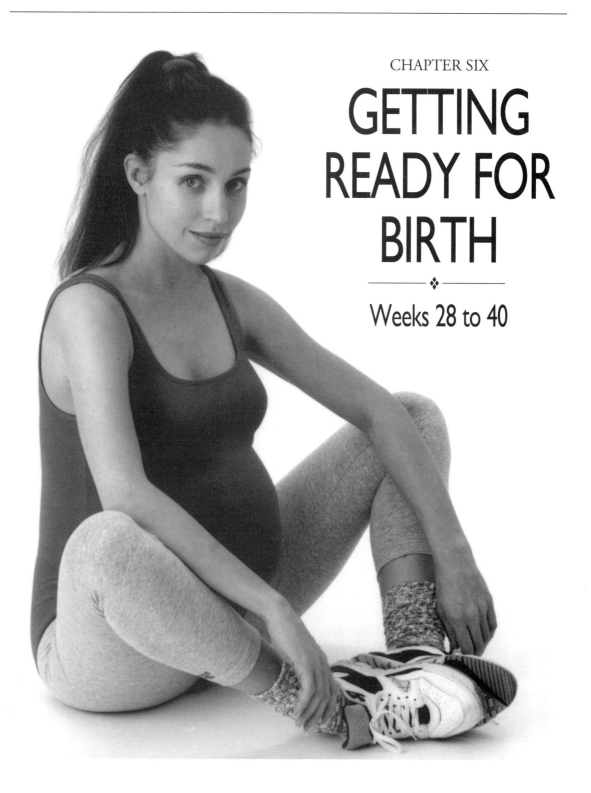

CHAPTER SIX

GETTING READY FOR BIRTH

❖

Weeks 28 to 40

THIS IS THE FINAL TRIMESTER. Your pregnancy is gradually drawing to a close, and soon you will be a mother! Up until now your thoughts have probably been focused on 'being pregnant', but now you are likely to find yourself thinking more and more about the birth itself – or, more to the point, wondering how much it is going to hurt!

Unfortunately, there is no straightforward answer to that question. Everyone's labour is different, and so is everyone's perception of pain. The only thing everyone is agreed on is that it really *is* all worthwhile!

Although there is no way of guaranteeing yourself a pain-free labour, you can do several things at least to make it easier.

WRITE A BIRTH PLAN

Thinking now about the sort of birth you want, and then putting your thoughts down on paper, is helpful in several ways. Firstly, it helps to focus your mind on what lies ahead. Think about pain relief and whether you want an epidural or not. Do you want to stay mobile during labour, or remain on the bed? Do you want an injection to speed up delivery of the placenta, or do you want to deliver it naturally? Would you rather tear a bit naturally than be given an episiotomy? Do you mind if there are students watching the birth? Do you want your baby cleaned up before you hold him? And so on.

Reading up about labour and birth will help you to prepare your answers – and prepare yourself. Remember, however, that you do not know what will happen 'on the day' or how you will feel, so do not make your plan dogmatic – be prepared to be flexible. An epidural may suddenly seem like a very good idea when your contractions are hotting up!

The plan also helps to prepare your birth partner. If he or she knows what you would like to happen, he or she can help you achieve that on the day. When you are concentrating on your contractions, you are not going to feel like chatting about your preferences. The midwife who delivers your baby will also find it useful to read your birth plan. It helps him or her to find out a bit about you without distracting you with questions.

Once you have written your plan, show it to a midwife or doctor, and ask for their comments – then do not forget to keep it with you when you go into labour!

LEARN TO RELAX

All the exercises in this book are ideal for teaching you more control of your body, but the pelvic floor and relaxation exercises are especially important. Whenever we become frightened or stressed the automatic reaction is to tense our muscles. Think about what you do when you are in a stressful situation. You probably grit your teeth, hunch your shoulders, clench your fists or get a tense neck. If you are in pain, this will only make the pain seem worse. Only by relaxing your muscles – and especially those areas prone to tension – will the pain seem easier to cope with.

When you go into labour, the contractions will get gradually stronger and more painful, but by relaxing your body you will stay more in control of the pain.

As you will have discovered in the relaxation sessions in this book, deep breathing helps your body unwind. By breathing in deeply through your nose and out through your mouth, until you feel as if every bit of air has left your body, your muscles will gradually relax. When you are pregnant you will hear a lot of talk about breathing exercises, but this is really the only 'exercise' you need to remember – it is that easy.

When you are in the second stage of labour, and your baby's head is about to be born, your ability to relax your body, and especially your pelvic floor, can make the difference between your perineum tearing badly or staying intact. As the head 'crowns' it is important that you stay in control and do not push – however great the urge. This enables the midwife to ease the head out slowly and gently, without your tearing. He or she will ask you to relax your pelvic floor muscles and make short, quick breaths outwards through your mouth ('panting'), to prevent you from pushing. The greater your body awareness is, the more you will be able to cope with this.

STAY MOBILE

The days when women gave birth flat on their backs with their legs in the air are, thankfully, disappearing fast, and the emphasis now is on staying mobile during labour and on freedom of birthing position.

The reason for this is obvious, if you think about it. If you are lying flat on your back on a bed, your baby has to fight hard against gravity in order to make his way down the birth canal. If you are upright, or at least your pelvis is, his or her journey into the world is made much easier.

It has also been proved that staying upright and on the move keeps your contractions going, and makes your labour more effective – and as anything that makes your labour more effective will also make it shorter and easier for you, it would seem well worth giving it a go!

Illustrated in this chapter are some positions that will be comfortable during labour, yet keep your body in a position which will encourage the labour to progress. The exercises you have been doing throughout your pregnancy will have kept you fit and strong, but walking and standing around will still get tiring after a while, and you may find that your back gets sore, too. Adopting one of these positions should soothe aches and pains slightly.

LEARN ABOUT LABOUR

The more you know about what is happening to your body and your baby during your labour, the less strange and frightening it will be. Your antenatal classes should be able to give you all the information you need and answer your questions, but you should also buy or borrow books from the library about labour and birth. If nothing else, remember one thing: contractions are your body's way of helping your baby down the birth canal – or, in other words, every contraction means your baby (and the end!) is getting a little bit closer. That should help you to think positively, and maybe even greet each contraction with a smile!

HAVE A SUPPORTIVE BIRTH PARTNER

Trends in childbirth change, and so do attitudes to having fathers at the birth. Whereas our fathers probably paced outside with a cigar while mum got on with it alone, it is now the norm for men to be there through thick and thin, shouting encouragement and even cutting the umbilical cord. That is all very well if your partner is the cheerleading type, but there are plenty of others who cannot even watch a birth on television, and have no intention of seeing the real thing. Certain bodies are now beginning to wonder if we have gone too far and are pushing our 'new men' too hard. If they are going to faint, be sick, or are simply terrified, maybe it is better that they do wait outside until the worst is over.

Do not assume that your partner is going to fall into either camp. Give him a chance to think about what he feels and then talk about it together. Think carefully about what you want, too. A lot of women decide that *they* would prefer their partner to be on the other side of the delivery-room door. Some do not like the idea of their partner seeing them in such an undignified state, others are worried that they will say something dreadful while in the thick of contractions, and many realize that if he is going to be there under duress, it is probably better that he is not there at all.

Whatever you both decide, respect one another's decision. From your point of view, you are going to need someone who will be a good support all the way through; someone who knows you well enough to interpret how you are feeling, and voice your wishes to others, and someone who will not mind if you shout at them a bit – manners do tend to disappear in the delivery room. If your partner is not going to be there, why not ask your mother, sister or a good friend instead?

Once you have decided who it is going to be, go through your birth plan with them and let them know how they can help you during labour. Sometimes just words of support, or a hand to hold, are enough. Other wome find they need someone to support the physically too, so that they can squat bend over for longer. And a partner wh good at massage or back rubbing is a bor

POSTURE

Posture at this stage in your pregnancy is more important than ever. You have got a big weight to carry now, and it is all out in front – it is hardly surprising that your centre of gravity changes. As before, take a long look at the way you stand in the mirror and go through the checkpoints given in Chapter 1. Christina, shown here, was due to have her baby the day these photos were taken – just look at the difference adopting good posture has on her overall shape.

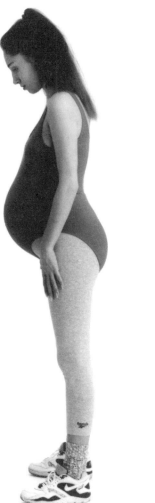

Bad

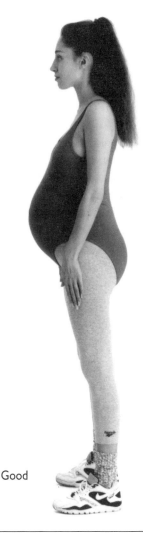

Good

POSITIONS FOR LABOUR

You may not be planning on having a completely natural childbirth, but you can still help
to make your labour more comfortable by using
certain positions. Practising these positions
while you are pregnant will not only help you
get used to how they feel, it will enable you to
stay in them for longer on the day, and make
your body stronger and more able to cope with
labour pain.

1 PELVIC TILT

Get on to all fours, with your knees slightly
more than hip-distance apart and your back
straight. Tighten your tummy muscles to protect your back.

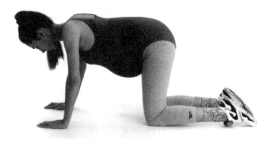

Now tuck your pelvis up and under, so that
your back rounds. Clench your buttock muscles
for a few seconds, then release them and return
to your start position, without letting your back
sink downwards. Try the same movement while
gently rocking your pelvis up and down. This
can be soothing during labour.

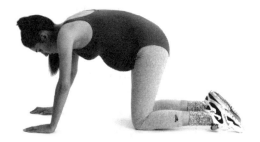

2 SQUATTING

Stand with your back long and straight and
your feet about 45cm (18in) apart. Tilt your
pelvis and tighten your stomach muscles. Squat
down as far as you comfortably can (but no
further than knee level), keeping your back
straight. You can lean against a wall for support
if it helps. Try to distribute your weight evenly
between your heels and toes. Hold for as long
as you feel comfortable, then come up again.
You should already be squatting like this whenever you need to pick up anything low.

Practise squatting as often as you can. It
makes your pelvis more flexible, relieves backache and will strengthen your thigh and back
muscles – useful for helping you support your
bump, and when in labour. You may even find
that you want to give birth in this position, so
the stronger your thighs are the better.

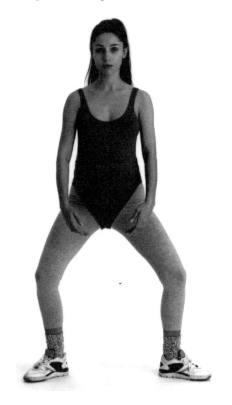

3 STANDING

Stand with your legs hip-distance apart, facing the back of a chair and rest your arms on it. Gently rock your pelvis from side to side, and back and forth, breathing steadily in through your nose and out through your mouth. Rocking the pelvis can be soothing during labour, and staying upright will help to keep your contractions coming and speed up labour.

4 SITTING

Sit astride a chair, with your legs wide apart, facing the back and lean over the back of the chair, resting your head on your arms or a cushion if you wish. Make sure your back is straight, then practise gentle, steady breathing, relaxing your body as much as possible. Breathe in through your nose and out through your mouth. When you want to sit down during labour, this is the best way to do it.

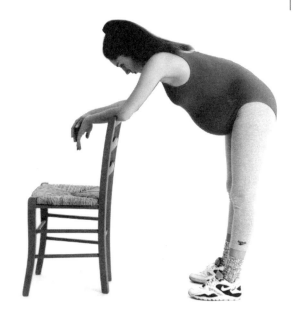

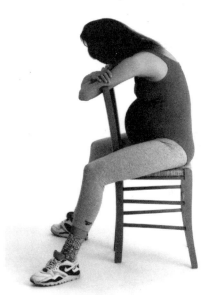

5 TAILOR SITTING

Sit on the floor with your legs out in front of you and your back straight. Think tall to lift yourself up out of your waist, and keep your shoulders down. Bend your knees so that you bring the soles of your feet together, then move them in towards your groin. Let your knees drop down towards the floor and breathe deeply. The more you practise this position, the closer to your groin your feet will go. Placing your hands on the floor behind you will help you ease your body forwards towards your heels to increase the stretch.

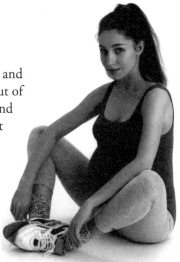

THE WORKOUT (A MOBILITY ROUTINE)

The term workout sounds a little strenuous for this stage of your pregnancy, but these simple exercises will keep you feeling fit and supple.

You will be feeling heavier and perhaps more tired now, especially as the big day approaches. However, there is no reason why you should not continue to exercise right up until you give birth – unless of course, you have been advised not to for a medical reason. Some days, however, you may feel somewhat lacking in energy. Do not worry. Why not do the warm-up routine to keep you mobile, and save the further stretches for another day?

TURN TO CHAPTER 1 FOR THE WARM-UP ROUTINE or listen to your tape, if you have recorded one. Note the following points before you start:

• Omit the hamstring stretch on your back. You can do a standing version instead.

• Take care when you do the hip circles that you do not arch your back.

• Maintain your pelvic tilt, and hold in your tummy muscles throughout to give your back extra protection.

• Use a chair for support when doing the side bends and upward reaches.

Now you are warmed up, you are ready to start.

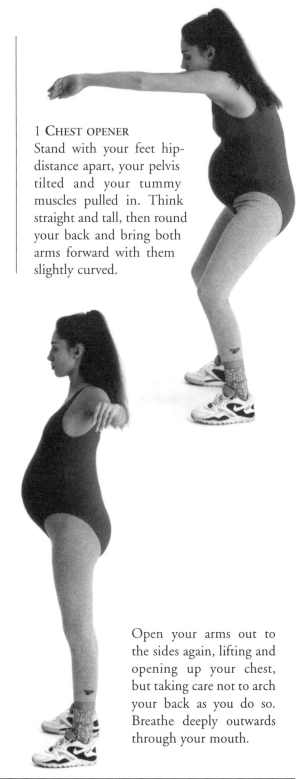

1 CHEST OPENER
Stand with your feet hip-distance apart, your pelvis tilted and your tummy muscles pulled in. Think straight and tall, then round your back and bring both arms forward with them slightly curved.

Open your arms out to the sides again, lifting and opening up your chest, but taking care not to arch your back as you do so. Breathe deeply outwards through your mouth.

2 ARM CIRCLES
Still standing straight, with one hand resting on your hip, lift the other arm forwards . . .

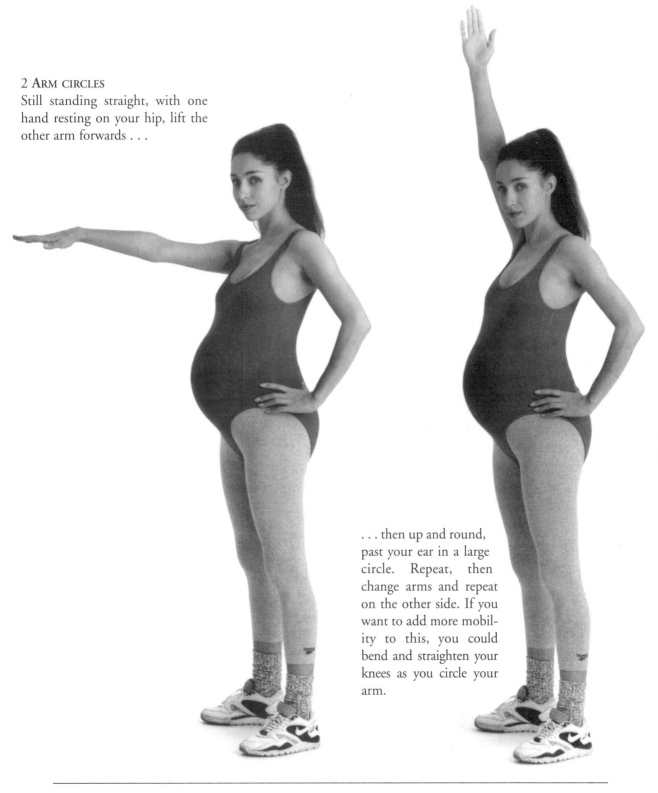

. . . then up and round, past your ear in a large circle. Repeat, then change arms and repeat on the other side. If you want to add more mobility to this, you could bend and straighten your knees as you circle your arm.

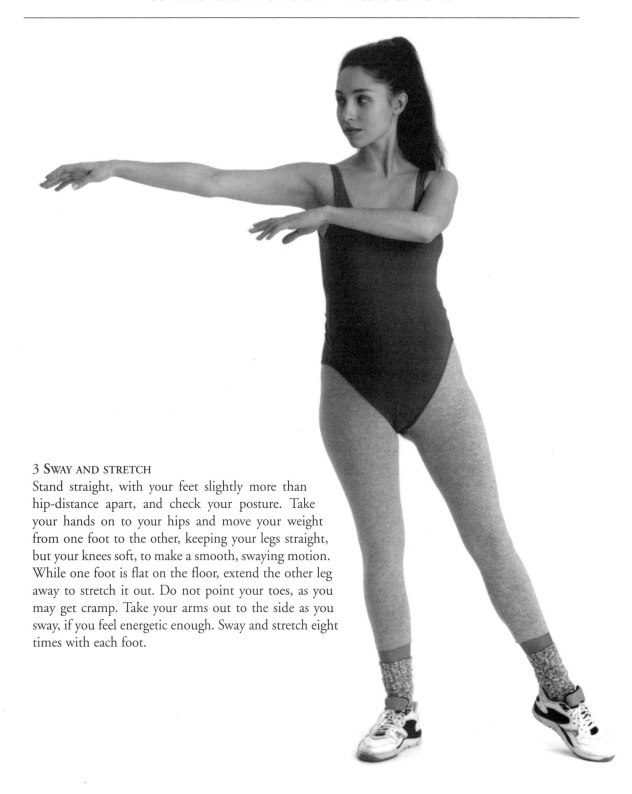

3 SWAY AND STRETCH

Stand straight, with your feet slightly more than hip-distance apart, and check your posture. Take your hands on to your hips and move your weight from one foot to the other, keeping your legs straight, but your knees soft, to make a smooth, swaying motion. While one foot is flat on the floor, extend the other leg away to stretch it out. Do not point your toes, as you may get cramp. Take your arms out to the side as you sway, if you feel energetic enough. Sway and stretch eight times with each foot.

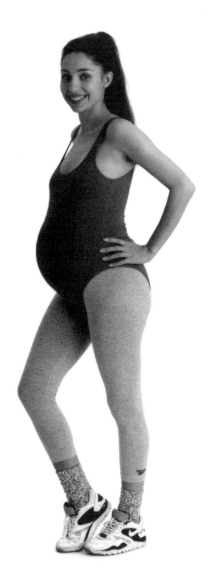

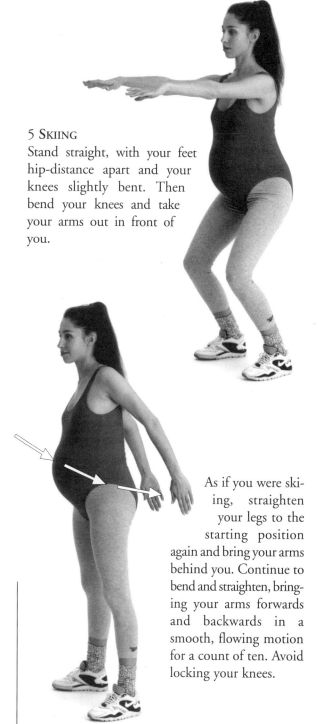

5 SKIING

Stand straight, with your feet hip-distance apart and your knees slightly bent. Then bend your knees and take your arms out in front of you.

As if you were skiing, straighten your legs to the starting position again and bring your arms behind you. Continue to bend and straighten, bringing your arms forwards and backwards in a smooth, flowing motion for a count of ten. Avoid locking your knees.

4 WALKING ON THE SPOT

With your back straight and your shoulders relaxed and down, begin to walk through your feet, from toe to heel, lifting your heels and transferring your weight from foot to foot. Put your hands on your hips or let your arms swing freely back and forwards if you wish, and keep a pelvic tilt throughout. Do not let yourself drop into your hips. Continue for about 30 seconds.

6 Leg curls

This exercises the buttocks and the backs of your thighs.

Stand holding on to a chair or the wall for extra support, either facing it or sideways on. Maintain a pelvic tilt. Keep your feet flat on the floor and your knees slightly apart and bent. Lift your right leg straight behind you (you will not be able to lift it very far).

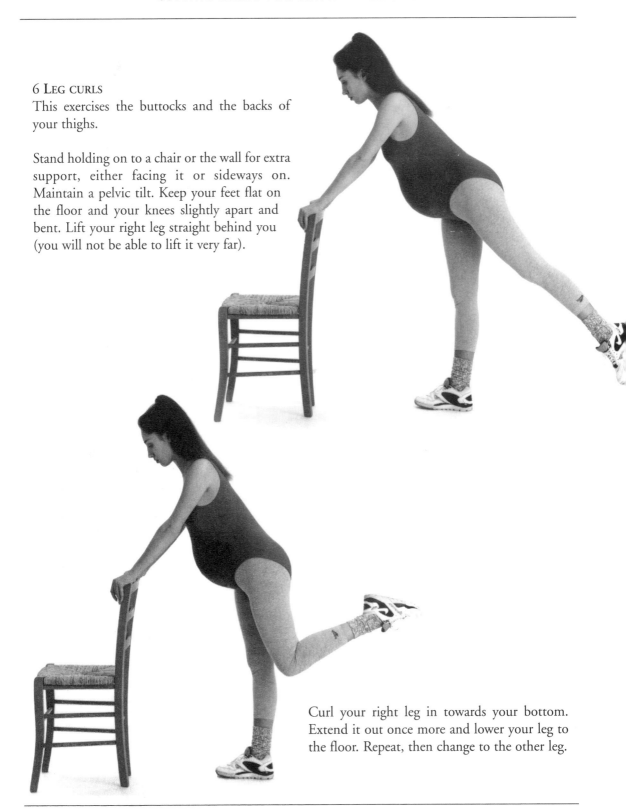

Curl your right leg in towards your bottom. Extend it out once more and lower your leg to the floor. Repeat, then change to the other leg.

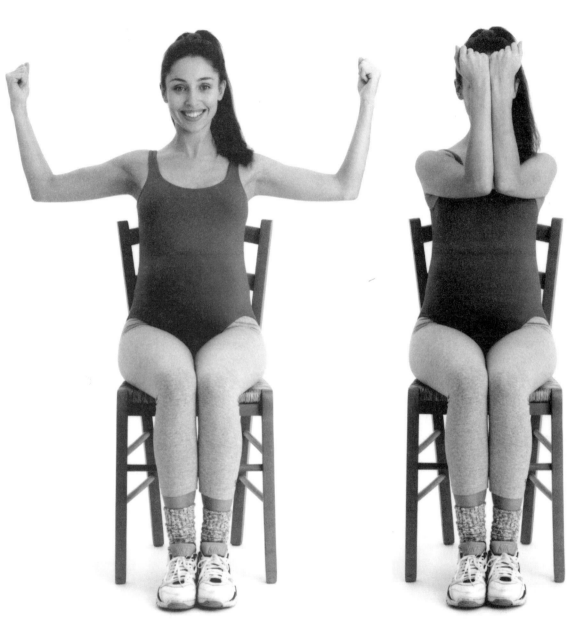

7 PECTORAL PRESSES

Sit comfortably, with your back lifted out of your hips and straight and your tummy muscles pulled in. With your arms out at your sides, bend your elbows at right angles.

Slowly press your elbows together in front of your chest and open out again. Work your muscles hard as if you were having to squeeze a ball in front of you. This works your chest as well as your arms. Repeat.

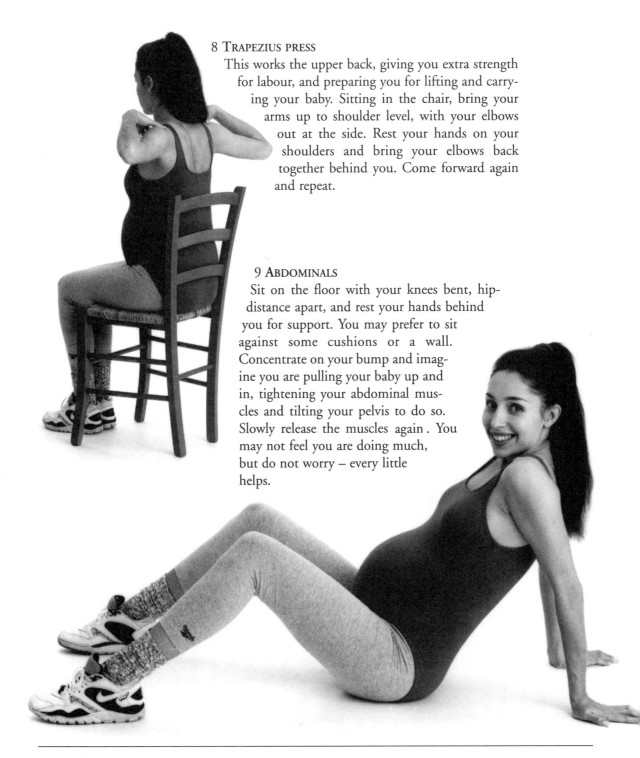

8 TRAPEZIUS PRESS

This works the upper back, giving you extra strength for labour, and preparing you for lifting and carrying your baby. Sitting in the chair, bring your arms up to shoulder level, with your elbows out at the side. Rest your hands on your shoulders and bring your elbows back together behind you. Come forward again and repeat.

9 ABDOMINALS

Sit on the floor with your knees bent, hip-distance apart, and rest your hands behind you for support. You may prefer to sit against some cushions or a wall. Concentrate on your bump and imagine you are pulling your baby up and in, tightening your abdominal muscles and tilting your pelvis to do so. Slowly release the muscles again. You may not feel you are doing much, but do not worry – every little helps.

Cool down

Hold the stretches for as long as is comfortable. A count of six to eight is fine.

Do not forget your pelvic floor exercises. You can do them while you are sitting for the cool down.

10 PECTORAL STRETCH
Carefully sit down in the tailor position or cross-legged and clasp your hands loosely behind your lower back, with your palms facing upwards. Bring your shoulder blades down and together, so that your elbows come closer and you can feel the stretch across your chest. Make sure that your lower back does not arch as you do this. Hold and then relax.

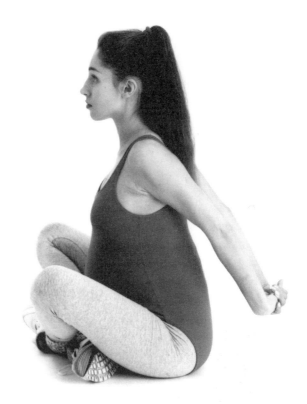

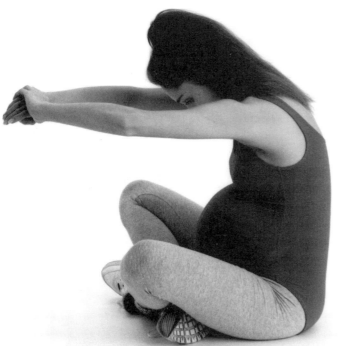

11 TRAPEZIUS STRETCH
Sitting in the same position, bring your arms in front of you and clasp your hands loosely together. Push away from you into your hands, so that you feel the stretch across your upper back. Hold and then relax.

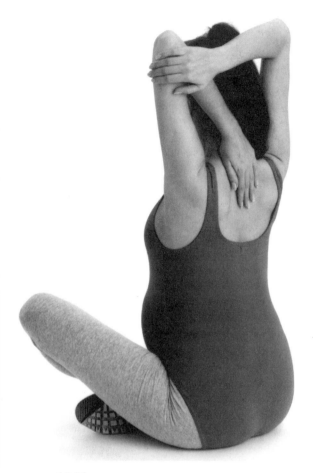

13 INSIDE THIGH STRETCH

Bring the soles of your feet together into the tailor position and gently move your knees outwards until you feel a stretch along the inside of your thighs. You may need to bring your legs closer into you in order to achieve this. By placing your hands behind your back, you can ease your body forwards into the stretch.

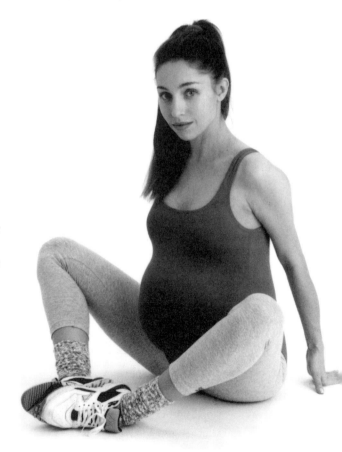

12 TRICEPS STRETCH

Circle both shoulders backwards a couple of times, then slowly lift one arm up above your head. Bend it at the elbow so that the lower half of your arm falls to your neck. Rest it there and gently use the other hand to support the arm as you stretch it. Hold, then gently release and change sides.

14 HAMSTRING STRETCH

Straighten out your left leg, keeping your left leg bent, with both slightly off-centre. Place your hands on the floor behind you for support and gently ease your body forward. Feel the stretch in the back of the straight leg. Hold the stretch, then repeat on the other side.

15 UPWARD REACH

Sitting cross-legged, your back straight and your tummy muscles pulled in, reach your left hand up above your head, lifting yourself up and out of your hips. Stretch up as high as is comfortable, hold it, then release and repeat on the other side.

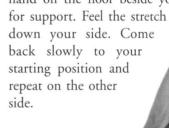

16 SIDE STRETCH

Sitting cross-legged, your back straight and your tummy muscles pulled in, reach your right hand up above your head and over to the other side, keeping your other hand on the floor beside you for support. Feel the stretch down your side. Come back slowly to your starting position and repeat on the other side.

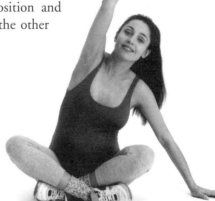

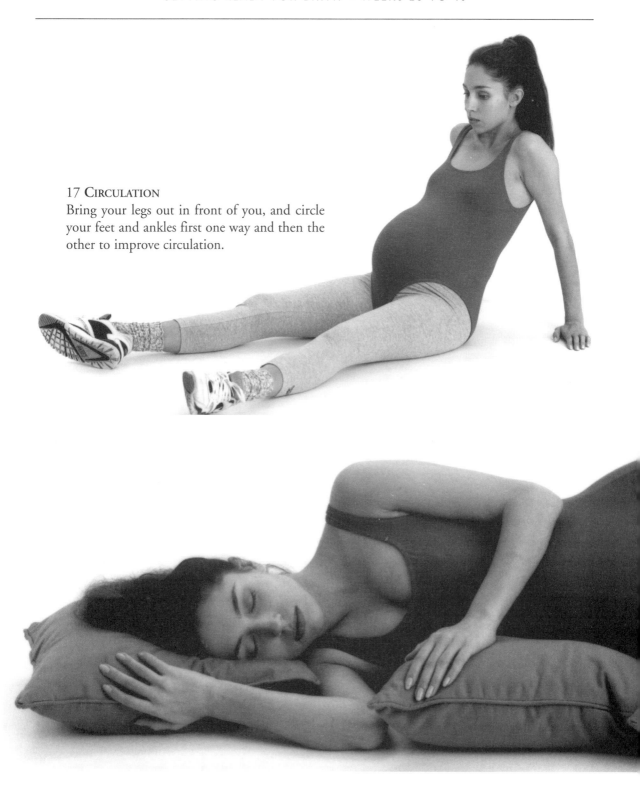

17 CIRCULATION
Bring your legs out in front of you, and circle your feet and ankles first one way and then the other to improve circulation.

18 RELAXATION

Learning how to relax your body is important during labour. Tension increases feelings of pain, and the more you can relax, reduce tension and breathe through contractions, the better you will cope with them. The relaxation exercises you have done in the workouts up to now will have developed your awareness of your body and how to relax the individual muscles in it, so take a few minutes every day to repeat them.

You are going to be much larger and heavier now and will need more rest, so do not fight it – relax! You will not have much time to lie back and close your eyes when the baby is born, so enjoy it now.

Follow the guidelines given in the workout in Chapter 5. You will feel more comfortable lying on your side supported by cushions, or perhaps sitting in a comfortable chair. Close your eyes and take as long as you like to unwind completely.

Congratulations – you have finished your workout.

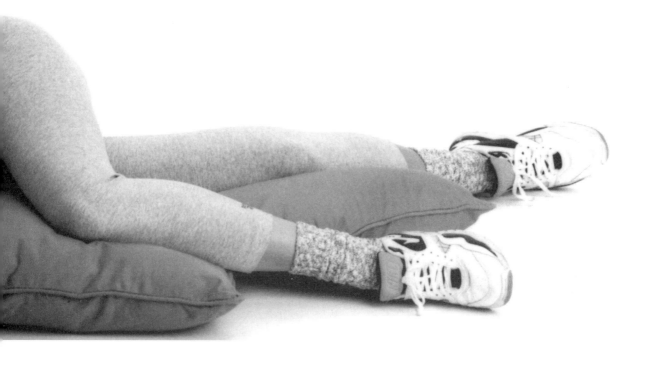

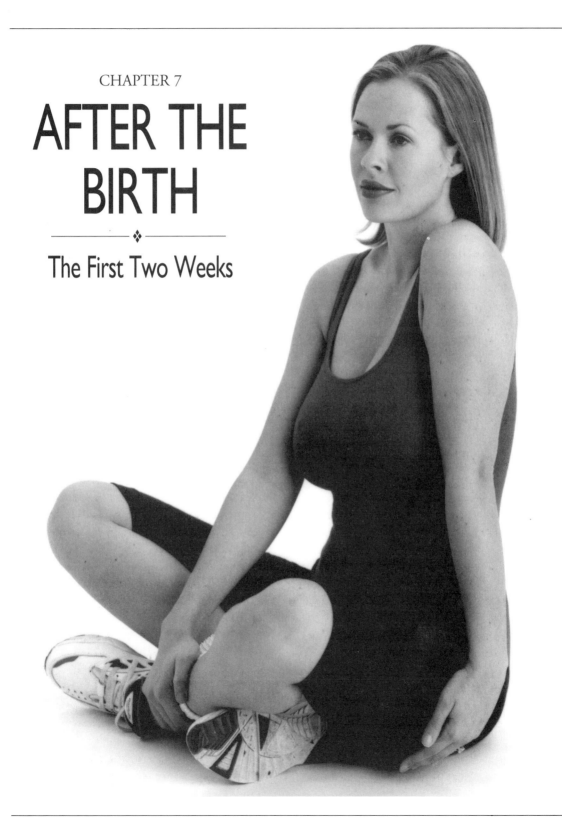

CHAPTER 7

AFTER THE
BIRTH

❖

The First Two Weeks

WELL DONE – you have given birth to a wonderful new baby! You deserve, and should, take it easy for a while now. Your body has had to work very hard to perform this amazing feat and it will take sometime for it to recover.

THE FIRST WEEK

How you feel at the moment will largely depend on how the birth went – some are undoubtedly harder than others, so do not feel you should be up and running around, simply because the woman in the bed next to you is. If the labour was very long, you had an episiotomy, or especially if you had a Caesarean, it will take a few days before you begin to feel anything like normal, and weeks or months before your body returns to its pre-pregnant state.

Take it easy

If you are in hospital, make the most of the opportunity to worry about nothing more than the care of yourself and your baby. Sleeping can be difficult in a noisy ward, but rest as much as you can. Your baby will probably be a bit sleepy for the first couple of days, so take your lead from her. If you are at home, resist the urge to get up and tidy, have constant visitors or generally rush around. Imagine that you are still in hospital, at least for five days after the birth, and give yourself time to get to know the new arrival too.

After an episiotomy

If you needed an episiotomy, or tore slightly to deliver your baby, you will be feeling rather sore. If you are in hospital, you will be given painkillers, and if you are at home, you can take paracetamol. Sitting on a rubber ring can make you a bit more comfortable, but you should not sit on it for too long as it will stop you healing as quickly.

Frozen peas are the answer to many a new mother's prayers. The same bag can be refrozen time after time – so long as you can identify it from the other peas in the freezer! Wrap it in a small towel or cloth and sit on it – or you could carry it around in your knickers. Again, you should not sit on the bag for extended periods, as this prevents the wound from healing as efficiently.

Have showers in preference to baths for the first few days if you can, as soaking the stitches for long periods of time is not advisable. If you do not have a shower, keep your baths short.

Often, the thought of the stitches is far worse than the reality. It might put your mind at rest to look at the area in the mirror.

After a Caesarean

A Caesarean scar is quite debilitating for a while, and you need to be more careful than other new mothers until six weeks after the birth. To begin with, getting up and about will be awkward. However, it is important that you do get out of bed as soon as possible, as it will get your circulation going and speed up your recovery. Hospital physiotherapists will be able to advise you on moving about carefully and the care of your scar, for both now and when you go home. Your relaxation and breathing techniques will stop you becoming tense with any pain and will help you to move more easily.

If you are keen to get back into shape quickly, you may feel frustrated that you cannot move around as much as other new mothers, but do not worry. You can still do the exercises given in these chapters, as long as you are careful with your technique and do not push yourself so much that you put a strain on your scar. You might want to cut out the gentle curl-ups for a few weeks and just do some static abdominal exercises. Wait until at least ten weeks after the birth before you perform any other sort of workout routine.

If you are breastfeeding your baby, you will need to adopt different feeding positions to other mothers. Using pillows for support will help, but you may find it most comfortable with both you and your baby lying on your sides. While you are in hospital, someone will be able to help you to find the most comfortable position.

Your scar will gradually become less sore and fade to a small white mark which will hardly be noticeable.

Food for thought

Now that you have had your baby, it is vital that you keep your strength up, so a healthy diet is just as important now as when you were pregnant. Breastfeeding demands a lot of energy and so eats up extra calories, but try to replenish those calories with nutritious food instead of naughty, sugar-filled snacks which provide 'empty calories', rather than nutrition.

Constipation can be a problem for new mothers, as labour tends to slow the passage of faeces through your bowels, and you may not have eaten properly for a couple of days. This, combined with worry about your stitches and feeling rather sore, can reduce the urge to 'go'. Eat a healthy diet, including plenty of fibrous foods such as cereal, beans, dried fruit and wholemeal bread, and drink plenty of water and some fruit juice.

If you are breastfeeding, it is best not to take laxatives, as they are passed on to your baby via your milk.

Breast or bottle?

You have to think about your baby's diet now, too! Basically this comes down to breast- or bottlefeeding. Nutritionally speaking, you cannot fault breastfeeding. Mother Nature gives your baby everything that she needs – and never runs out. The antibodies in your milk also help to protect your baby from disease and allergies, such as asthma and eczema. So, if you have a history of such allergies in your family, you will be giving your baby the best start in life. Not only that – breastfeeding helps you get back into shape more quickly!

Formula milk can never match all this goodness, however hard the manufacturers try. However, some women prefer bottlefeeding because they feel it is better suited to their lifestyle. Breastfeeding can also be hard work initially, as you and your baby settle into a routine. The choice is yours, so choose whichever makes you feel happiest – after all, a happy you means a contented baby.

Mind and soul

The first week after the birth can be quite a shock, both physically and psychologically. The birth may not have gone as you expected and you probably did not realize how tired – and perhaps sore – you would feel. Even just the reality of having a baby to look after can be quite daunting. When you do not feel on top form, it is natural to want someone to look after and pamper you, so it can be difficult to accept that you have to look after the baby instead. Although people obviously have your interests at heart too, the baby is often the focus of their attention, and that can be hard to deal with when you are feeling low.

Do not feel guilty about these feelings; they

are completely natural and nothing to worry about. Your body is having to adjust to its pre-pregnant state and, once again, your hormones are adjusting too, leaving you feeling miserable and weepy from time to time. You may find you are especially tearful two or three days after the birth, when your milk 'comes in'. Have a good cry whenever you feel like it: no-one will blame you. The 'baby blues' are a commonly recognized problem.

The pelvic floor

Your cervix and vagina have, not surprisingly, been stretched considerably and your pelvic floor muscles will be soft and slack. Your cervix will firm up by itself in a week or so, but your pelvic floor needs some help from you. You can, and should, start doing your pelvic floor exercises again as soon as 24 hours after the birth, building up to five contractions about ten times a day. Why not do them every time you change your baby's nappy, and every time you have a cup of tea or coffee? Remember: if you do not do them, you run the risk of suffering from stress incontinence in the future, and your sex life may not be so satisfying. If you have had an episiotomy, pelvic floor exercises will also speed up healing.

THE WORKOUT

Do not panic: you are not expected to don your leotard and do a full workout straight after having the baby! However, it is important that you keep as mobile as possible and do a few basic exercises. These can easily be done while you are in hospital, simply lying on your bed.

Check your posture too, ideally in front of a mirror if you have access to one. During pregnancy, your body could adapt slowly to the change in weight and centre of gravity, but now

your baby has been born, it has to suddenly adjust to its pre-pregnant state. Your body may feel strange for the first few days, but if you keep checking that your posture is correct, it will prevent you straining your joints and muscles. Go back to Chapter 1 if you need a refresher on how to stand properly.

IF YOU HAVE HAD CAESAREAN, RE-READ THOSE SECTIONS BEFORE STARTING THE WORK-OUT.

Nicky had her baby 12 weeks ago, and she is already getting back into shape nicely. She is breastfeeding her baby, so her breasts are still quite heavy. Notice how good posture flattens her stomach and makes her look trimmer.

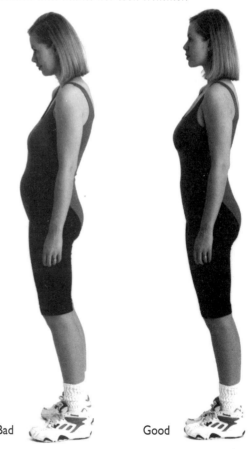

Bad   Good

The first 48 hours

This is a good time to start on your pelvic floor exercises again. You will not feel much to begin with, but the strength will soon come back.

1 TESTING YOUR ABDOMINALS

Your longitudinal abdominal muscles nearly always separate towards the end of pregnancy, to make room for your baby. You can gauge how well they are getting back into shape after the birth by checking regularly to see how the gap is closing up, although you have to make your muscles work quite hard in order to feel them at first.

Lie on your back with your knees bent. Pull your abdominal muscles in, lift up your head and shoulders, and stretch one arm hard down towards your feet. Put the fingers of your other hand in the centre of your stomach, just below your tummy button and feel for the gap in your muscles.

Do not panic if it seems very wide. Most people will have a gap at least two fingers wide, and a lot of women will have one three to four fingers wide. Eventually the gap will become so small that you will only be able to insert the tip of one finger.

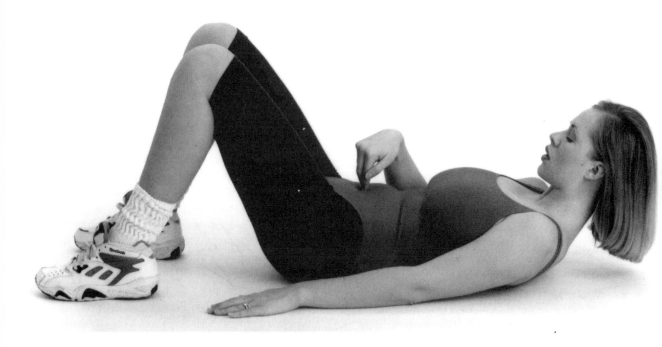

2 ABDOMINAL EXERCISE

This will help you relax, as well as toning your abdominals and improving your circulation. You can do this exercise in hospital, on the bed, with your baby next to you if you like.

Lie on your back with your knees bent. Breathe in slowly through your nose, then breathe out again through parted lips and draw in your abdominal muscles, pushing your back down into the bed and tilting your pelvis. Hold for a count of four and gently release. Continue to breathe like this to help you relax.

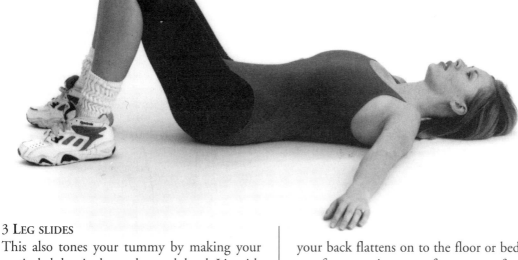

3 LEG SLIDES

This also tones your tummy by making your vertical abdominal muscles work hard. Lie with your knees bent and your feet flat on the floor or bed. Blow out and tighten your abdominals, while tilting your pelvis so that the hollow of your back flattens on to the floor or bed. Slide one foot at a time away from you as far as you can without allowing your back to arch. Breathe in, blow out and slowly draw your foot in again. Repeat five times.

To begin with, your back will arch when your feet are only a few inches away. This is because your abdominal muscles have been weakened. In time, you will be able to straighten and bend your legs completely.

4 FOOT CIRCULATION
This is especially beneficial if you are immobilized in bed after the birth. Lie with your legs straight and feet together. Briskly flex your feet up and down at the ankle for about 30 seconds. Move your feet apart slightly and circle your feet round in each direction: 20 times to the left, 20 times to the right.

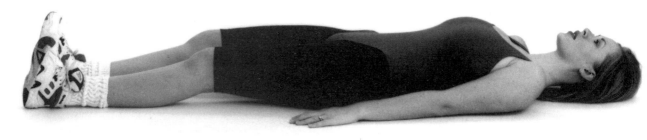

A week later – at home

Continue the first 48 hour exercises, but add the following:

ABDOMINALS AND WAIST
You can improve the tone of your tummy muscles by simply pulling them in, holding them for a count of four (continuing to breathe), and then releasing them slowly and with control. Do this any time you remember to, in any position.

1 CURL-UPS
Lie on your back on the floor, with your knees bent and feet flat on the floor. Tilt your pelvis as before and, keeping the tummy tight, raise your head, and possibly your shoulders (depending on how strong your muscles are), off the floor, while sliding your hands up your thighs towards your knees. Do not allow your tummy muscles to bulge as you do this. Repeat ten times. Avoid this exercise if you have had a Caesarean.

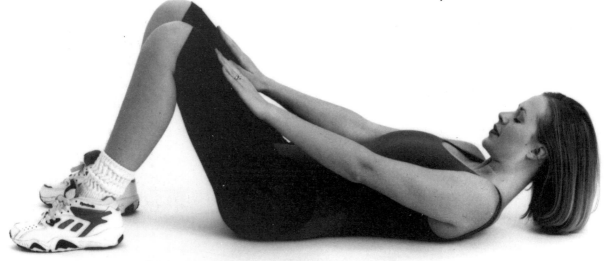

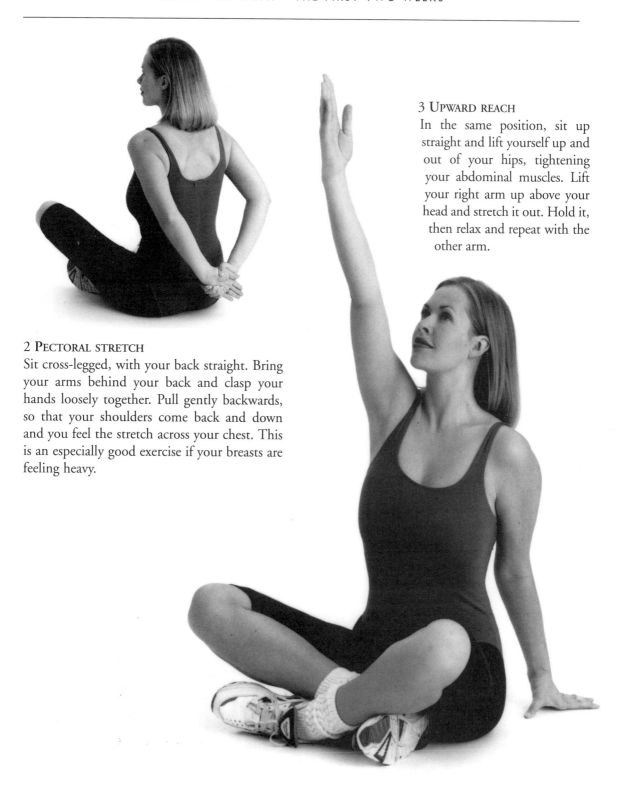

3 UPWARD REACH

In the same position, sit up straight and lift yourself up and out of your hips, tightening your abdominal muscles. Lift your right arm up above your head and stretch it out. Hold it, then relax and repeat with the other arm.

2 PECTORAL STRETCH

Sit cross-legged, with your back straight. Bring your arms behind your back and clasp your hands loosely together. Pull gently backwards, so that your shoulders come back and down and you feel the stretch across your chest. This is an especially good exercise if your breasts are feeling heavy.

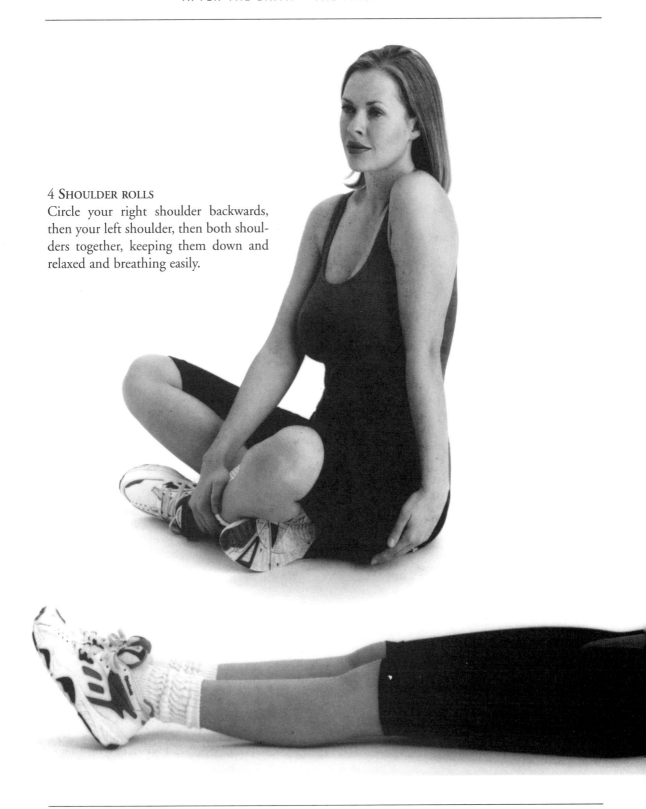

4 SHOULDER ROLLS

Circle your right shoulder backwards, then your left shoulder, then both shoulders together, keeping them down and relaxed and breathing easily.

5 RELAXATION

It is important to take time to relax now. Your body needs time to recover from the birth, and you will be busy each day (and night!) looking after and feeding your baby. Whenever you get the chance, stretch out and relax, using the techniques given in Chapters 3, 5 and 6.

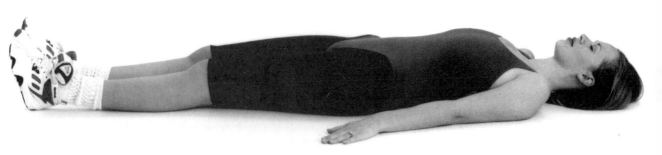

6 FULL BODY STRETCH

After you have relaxed, stretch your arms up as high above your head as you can, and extend your feet as far as possible in the opposite direction. Enjoy the stretch. Hold it, then relax.

Well done! You have already taken the first step towards regaining your figure. Repeat these gentle exercises whenever you get the opportunity.

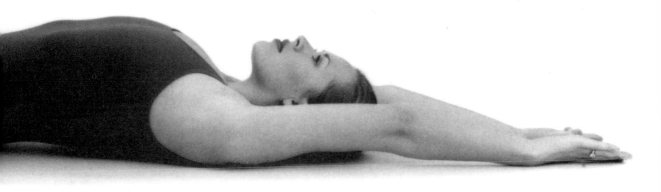

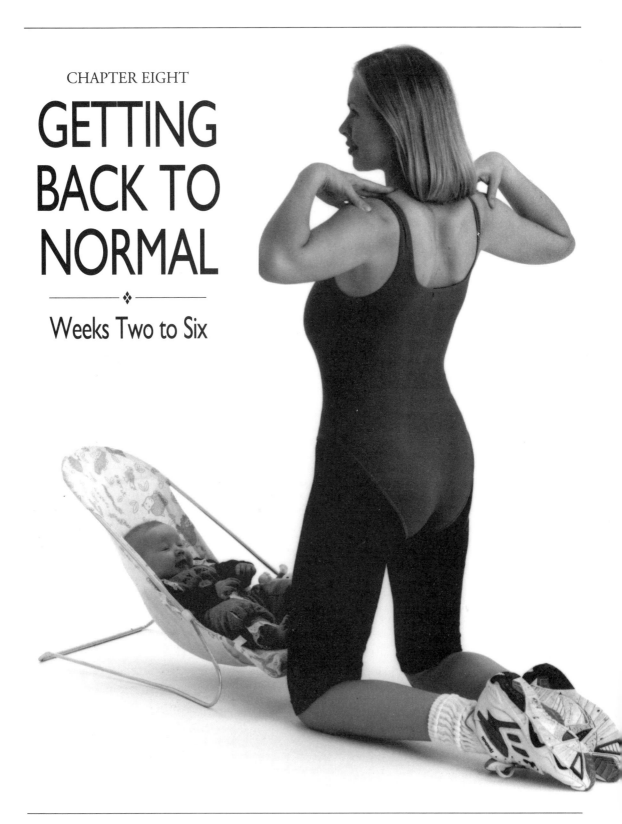

CHAPTER EIGHT

GETTING BACK TO NORMAL

❖

Weeks Two to Six

THE FIRST SIX WEEKS after the birth of your baby are a time of change for you, in all respects. Your body will be getting back to normal in some ways, but may still not feel like your own. Episiotomy and Caesarean scars will still be making their presence felt (although less so as time goes on), and if you are breastfeeding your breasts may seem overwhelming at times! Once your milk comes in they will expand considerably and will need the support of a good nursing bra. And, if they get overfull, they will have the habit of leaking or even spurting out the excess milk.

Do not expect your energy to return quickly. Your body has a lot to cope with, and you should rest as much as possible in order to allow it to recover. This can be difficult when you are at home, but just concentrate on yourself and the baby, and leave any chores to someone else, or until you feel better. Doing the gentle exercises in the workout in this chapter will actually help to give you a bit more energy, so do try to do them regularly, even if you do feel tired – but obviously do not push yourself too hard.

BACK BASICS

While you were pregnant you were probably given plenty of advice and warnings about straining your back, but it is just as applicable even now that you have had your baby. In fact, backache is one of the most common problems encountered in the early months after the birth. Your joints and ligaments are still looser than normal as a result of the hormonal changes in your body, and they will need some time to recover. Until then, you should continue to lift carefully (see page 37) and get up and down on to the floor as you did while you were pregnant (see page 38). Try to pick up and carry your baby without arching or straining your

back and, when you feed, choose a firm, upright chair and support yourself and your baby well with cushions. Remember to bring your baby to you, rather than bending over to your baby.

The exercises in the workout in this chapter will encourage good posture and help strengthen your tummy muscles to support your back. As ever, KEEP A CAREFUL EYE ON YOUR EXERCISE POSITION, TO MAKE SURE YOU ARE DOING IT CORRECTLY AND MAINTAINING GOOD POSTURE.

GOING HOME

Leaving hospital affects all women differently. Some cannot wait to be left to their own devices and get a decent rest away from the heat, light and chatter. Others feel safe and secure in hospital and are worried that they will not be able to cope with their baby by themselves when they go back home. Do not worry. You will never be left completely to your own devices, and further help is always available if you ask for it. Your doctor will know that you have been discharged and will probably arrange a home visit, as will your health visitor. Community midwives can also come in and make sure that you and the baby are settling in well, feeding is successful and so on.

Organizations such as the National Childbirth Trust in the UK also offer postnatal support on a local level. In addition, try to arrange for your partner to have some holiday when you come home from hospital, so that he can help out – perhaps your mother or a friend could come to stay for a while, too.

MORE THAN THE BLUES

For some women, the hormonal changes and the pressure of the new responsibility is all too much and they feel that they simply cannot cope. One in ten women will get the baby blues (see Chapter 7), but for one in 1,000, it goes beyond mere blues and is diagnosed as postnatal depression.

The earlier this is recognized and treated, the quicker the recovery – so if you feel out of control in any way, do talk about it to your doctor. The symptoms vary from person to person, but may include the following: lack of self esteem, feelings of guilt, obsessional thoughts, hopelessness, lack of appetite or interest in life, panic attacks and sleeping problems. Your doctor will probably prescribe anti-depressants for a while, and counselling if necessary. You *will* get better, given time.

YOUR PARTNER'S NEEDS

When you have got a new baby, and are feeling a bit overwhelmed by it all, it can put a strain on your relationship with your partner – at a time when everyone else is expecting you to be feeling even closer than before. For some people, a baby really does seem to bring them closer together, but plenty of others find that it puts an extra strain on the relationship. Adjusting to your new family takes time and requires a bit of effort.

It is true that you have got a lot on your plate at the moment, but try to see your partner's side, too. He may be feeling somewhat excluded from everything that is going on, especially if he is out at work all day and you are breastfeeding your baby. You are establishing a routine during the day which he has to try to adapt to when he comes home at night.

Try to include him in looking after the baby as much as you can, and do not criticize his efforts – you fumbled with your first nappies too, remember! Perhaps bathtime each evening could be his special time with the baby.

Do not forget that you are still a couple, too. It is very easy to get wrapped up in your baby's needs, to such an extent that you forget about your partner's. Make time to sit and cuddle or talk, or simply do some of the things you used to do together. You may not feel ready for sex yet, but try at least to share some quiet, intimate moments.

YOUR BABY'S NEEDS

In the determination to become supermum, we often exhaust ourselves by doing more than is really necessary. In the months to come your baby will begin to need extra stimulation, but at this early stage you need not feel you should be doing things to encourage her development every waking moment. All she needs from you now is warmth, food and plenty of love. Establishing feeding properly, keeping her room at the right temperature (about 18–19°C/ 64–66°F), keeping her clean and attending to her whenever she seems upset, is all that is required for now – as well as plenty of cuddles, of course!

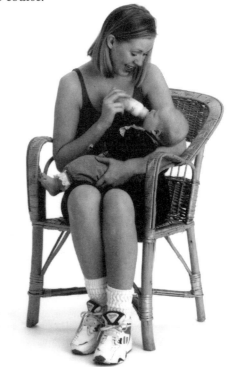

THE HEALTH VISITOR IN THE UK

Until you became pregnant, you had probably never even heard of health visitors. Hopefully, however, your health visitor made him or herself known to you when you became pregnant and you are now aware of the function he or she performs. From now on, your health visitor can play as large and important a part in caring for your family's health as you want him or her to. He or she will have a particular interest in the progress that your baby makes, but will also be concerned with the whole family's well-being, and can be a source of information and advice on most family concerns.

In the first few months after the birth of your baby, the health visitor can be most reassuring and helpful. He or she will hold a regular clinic locally, where you can take your baby to be weighed and measured and also ask any questions you have about feeding or your baby's general health. A lot of health visitors were once midwives and know a lot about caring for babies; however, they will always refer you to your doctor if they feel it is necessary. He or she will also know about other national and local support groups if you have any other particular problems. Make the most of these clinics – every new mother needs this kind of back-up.

YOUR BABY'S HEALTH

Your baby will have been thoroughly checked to make sure that she was fit and well when she was born, and again before she left hospital. But the check-ups do not end there. Everyone is as anxious as you are that she continues to progress as she should, and reviews are arranged for ten days, six weeks and seven or eight months after the birth. Make the most of these checks. By having your baby seen regularly by the professionals, you can be sure that any problems that do arise will be treated quickly.

Usually, in the UK, your family doctor or the clinical medical officer at the community health clinic will do the six-week check on your baby, while the health visitor sees her when she is seven months old.

You are likely to be given a Personal Child Health Record Book to keep at home and take with you whenever your child sees a health professional. Your health visitor, doctor and nurse will fill it in whenever relevant, so that you have a record of your baby's immunizations, weight, height and what happened at the check-ups or appointments, as well as medical information and advice. This book will tell you what to expect at each check-up.

However, no two babies are the same and they all progress at different rates, so do not worry too much if your baby does not seem to be doing everything they are checking for. However, if you are worried about anything, do mention it – the professionals rely on information from you, too.

THE WORKOUT

You can begin to exercise slightly more in earnest now, as long as you feel up to it. If you have had a Caesarean, wait until you have had your six-week check-up before you start these exercises, and do not join any class that is not specifically designed for postnatal exercise until at least ten weeks after the birth, as the abdominal exercises will put too much strain on your scar.

Repeat the exercises about five times each if you can. Set yourself a realistic goal and gradually increase the repetitions over the weeks.

Your baby will probably enjoy sitting and watching you exercising, so why not let her join in the fun. You will be setting her a great example!

BEFORE YOU START, TURN TO CHAPTER 1 AND FOLLOW THE POSTURE CHECK AND WARM-UP SEQUENCE AS USUAL.

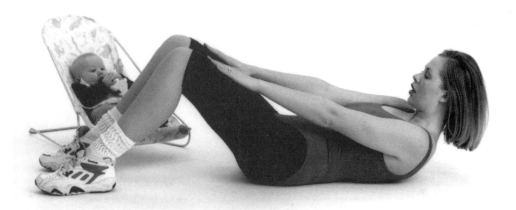

1 CURL-UPS

Lie on the floor with your knees bent and your feet flat on the floor. Tilt your pelvis, pulling in your abdominals, so that your back is flat on the floor, then blow out and slowly curl your head and shoulders up, bringing your hands up your thighs to your knees. Do not let your tummy muscles bulge outwards. Lower yourself slowly to the floor again. Repeat five times if you can, increasing as you grow stronger. If you cross your arms over your chest as you come up, it will make your muscles work even harder, but breastfeeding mums may have difficulties with this!

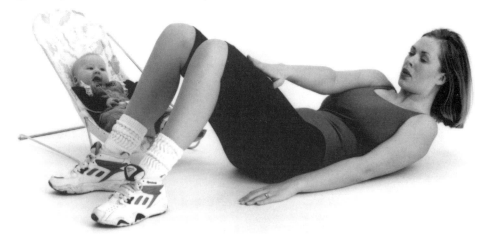

2 CURL-UP AND TWIST

Lying on the floor as before, contract your abdominal muscles then, blowing out, lift your head and shoulders off the ground and stretch your right hand across towards your left knee. Bring your shoulder, not just your arm, up and round, so that your upper body twists over. This exercises the oblique abdominal muscles. You will find that you will be able to curl higher as you get stronger, but do not push it now. Repeat five times on each side if you can, increasing the number of repetitions as you feel stronger.

Staying in the same position as for the last exercise, do some pelvic floor exercises. The more you practise them, the more you will be able to feel them working and the muscles becoming stronger.

3 WAIST WORK

In the same position, with your pelvic tilt maintained and your stomach muscles tightened, reach out and slide your left hand down towards your left foot, bending at the waist. Return to the starting position. Repeat to the other side, then repeat the sequence five times.

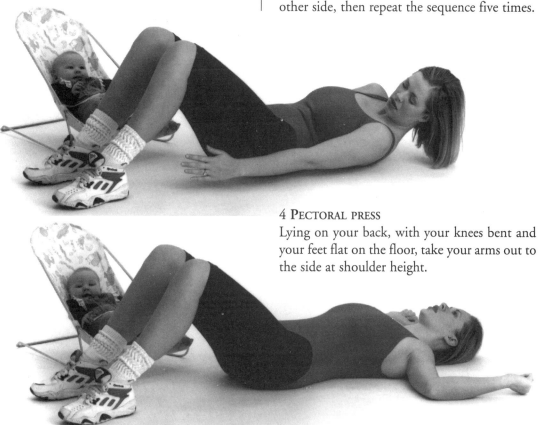

4 PECTORAL PRESS

Lying on your back, with your knees bent and your feet flat on the floor, take your arms out to the side at shoulder height.

Bend your arms up at right angles and slowly raise them up in front of your chest. Try to press your elbows together. Lower your arms slowly again, taking care that you do not allow your back to arch. Repeat five times.

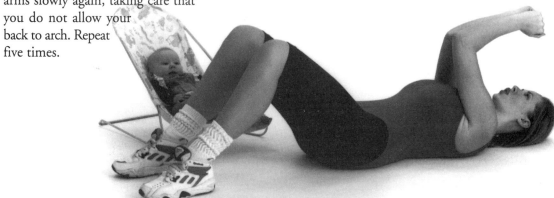

5 HIP HITCHES

Kneel on all fours, with your back straight and your legs hip-distance apart. Pull in your abdominal muscles and bring your hips round to the left and then to the right, so that you can feel the movement in your waist and abdominals. Repeat.

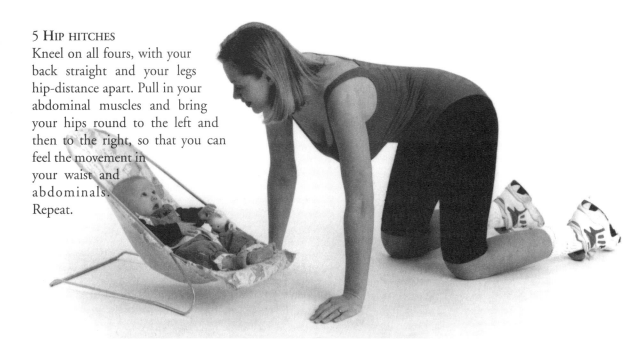

6 PELVIC ROCK

Kneel on all fours, with your back straight. Adopt a pelvic tilt, contract your abdominal and buttock muscles, and arch your back as you breathe out. Feel the stretch for a count of four, then release your back and your muscles gradually and come back to your starting position. Repeat the exercise again, feeling the rocking of your pelvis. This is great for relieving backache, too.

7 LEG RAISES

Stand facing a chair, holding the back for support, and tilt your pelvis. Keep your feet flat on the floor, your knees slightly apart and bent, and your back straight. Extend one leg out behind you, in a continuous line with your back. Lift and lower that leg, taking care that your back stays straight. Keeping your tummy muscles pulled in will help to protect your back. Repeat with the other leg.

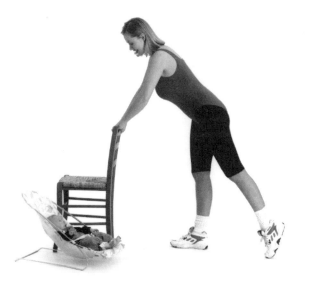

8 LEG CURLS

In the same starting position as before, slowly slide one foot back, until the knee is bent more and the toes of that foot rest behind on the floor.

Now lift that foot up towards your bottom, keeping your pelvis tilted and your back as straight as possible. Lower your foot again and bring it back to the start position. Repeat the sequence. You should feel the back of your thigh tighten. Then repeat with the other leg.

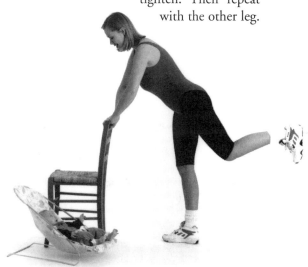

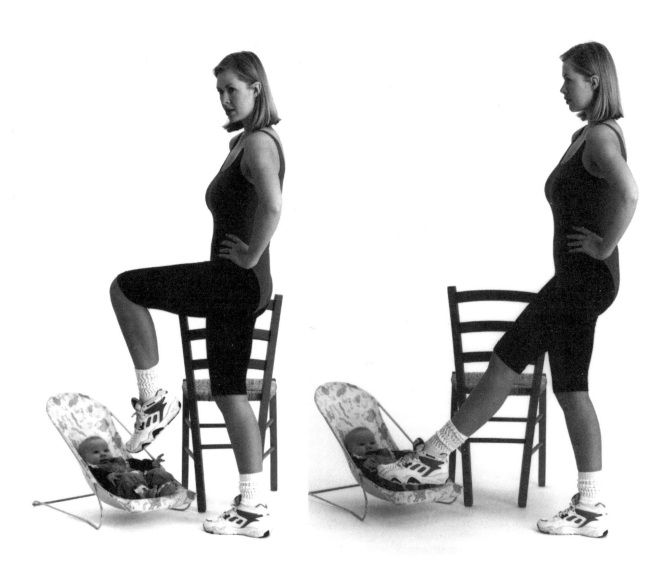

9 LEG EXTENSIONS

This exercises the front of your thigh. Stand holding on to your chair with one hand for support and check your posture. Tighten your abdominal muscles and lift your left knee up in front of you, keeping your back straight and your pelvis tilted.

Now slowly extend that leg in front of you before bringing it back to the starting position and repeating the sequence. Repeat with the other leg.

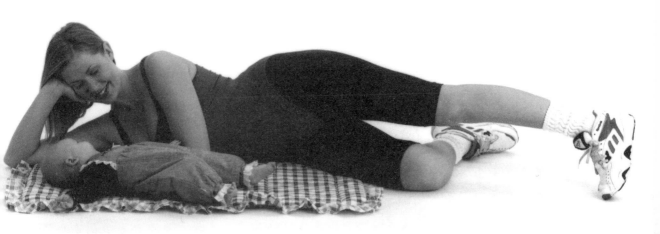

10 HIPS AND THIGHS

Lie on your left side, with your underneath leg bent and your top leg straight, and your head resting on your arm. Bring your other arm in front of you for support and look down the line of your body to your toes. Your shoulders, hips, knees and toes should be in a straight line. Do not lock your knees.

Pull in your abdominal muscles firmly and lift your right leg up in the air, keeping your toes facing forwards and the side of your leg facing the ceiling. Do not let your body rock backwards or forwards. Lower your leg again and repeat, before changing sides.

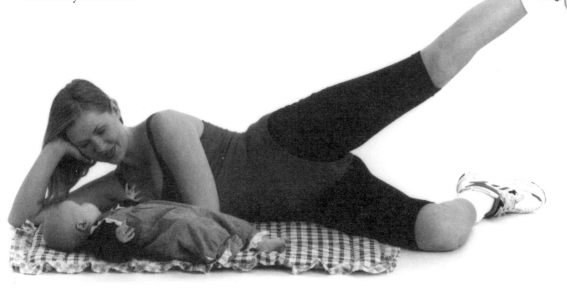

11 TRAPEZIUS PRESS

Kneel down and take your elbows out at shoulder height. Bring your hands up to rest on your shoulders, then push your elbows gently back towards the centre of your back. Bring them forwards again and repeat the sequence.

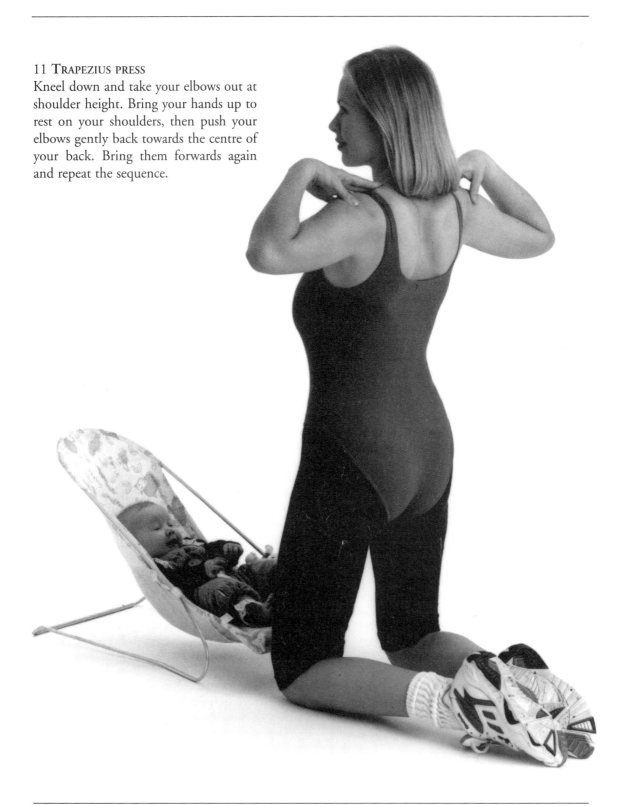

Cool down

Hold each stretch for as long as feels comfortable – a count of six to eight is fine.

12 PECTORAL STRETCH

Stand up and bring your arms behind you, clasping your hands loosely. Pull your arms gently backwards until you feel the stretch across your chest. Hold it and then release.

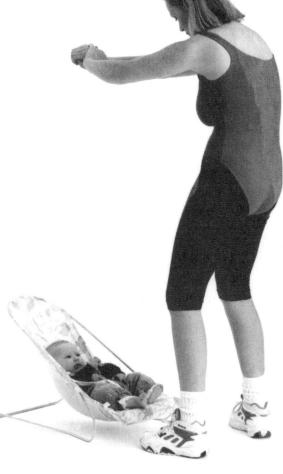

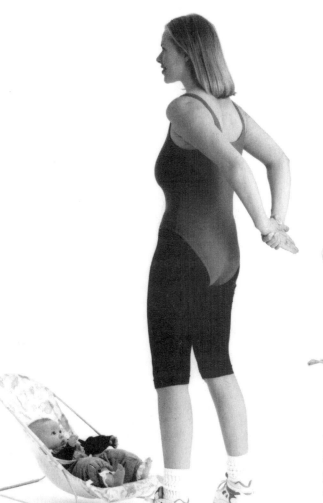

13 TRAPEZIUS STRETCH

Standing upright, take your arms in front of you and clasp your hands loosely. Pull your arms gently away from you, until you feel the stretch across your upper back. Hold, then relax.

14 TRICEP STRETCH

Take your left arm up and reach behind your back, using your right hand on the left elbow to ease the arm gently further down your back. Feel the stretch down the tricep, hold. Release the arm and repeat on the other side.

15 QUADRICEP STRETCH

Using your chair for support, stand upright, with your feet hip-distance apart, tilt your pelvis and bend your left leg up behind you. Clasp the foot with your left hand and use it to ease the leg closer to your bottom. Make sure your back is straight and your pelvis is tilted. Feel the stretch down the front of your thigh. Hold, then release the leg and repeat on the other side.

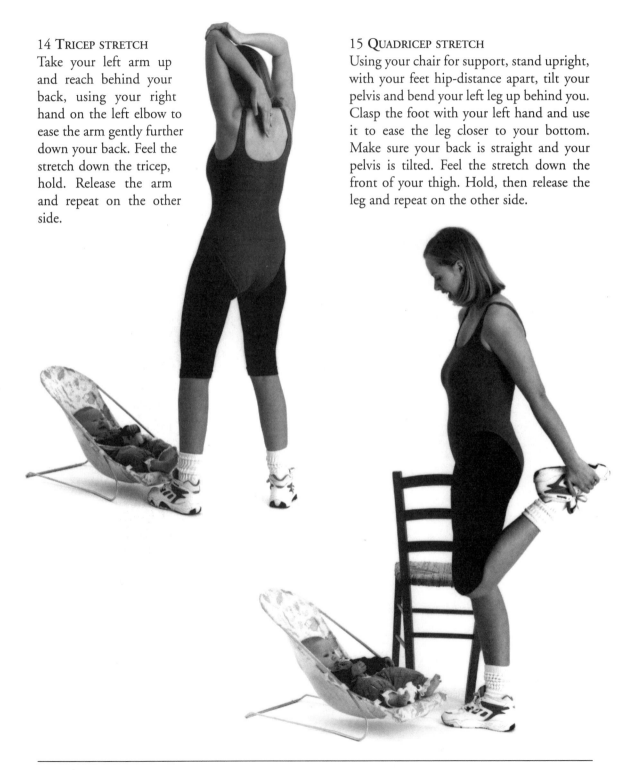

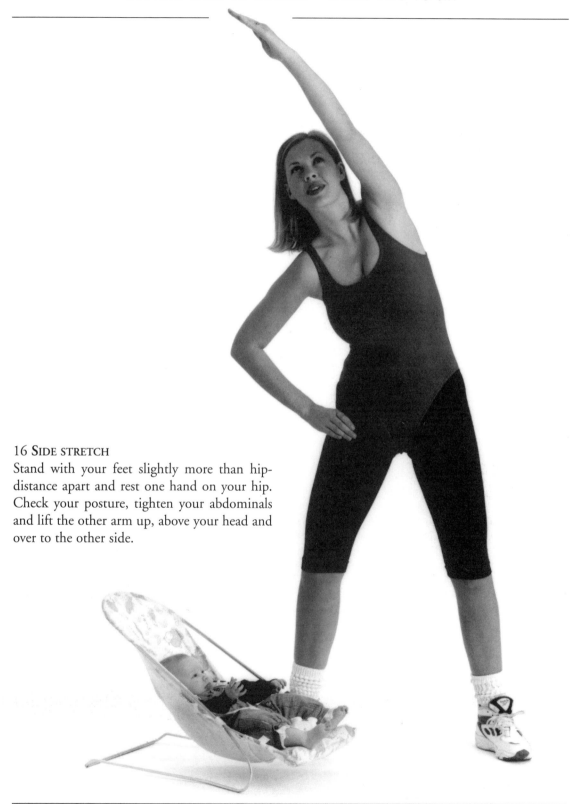

16 SIDE STRETCH

Stand with your feet slightly more than hip-distance apart and rest one hand on your hip. Check your posture, tighten your abdominals and lift the other arm up, above your head and over to the other side.

17 HAMSTRING STRETCH

Lie on your back with your knees bent and your feet flat on the floor. Lift one leg and bring it up towards you, bending at the knee. Take hold of your calf and gently ease the leg a little closer towards you, until you feel the stretch down your hamstring. Hold, then relax and repeat with the other leg.

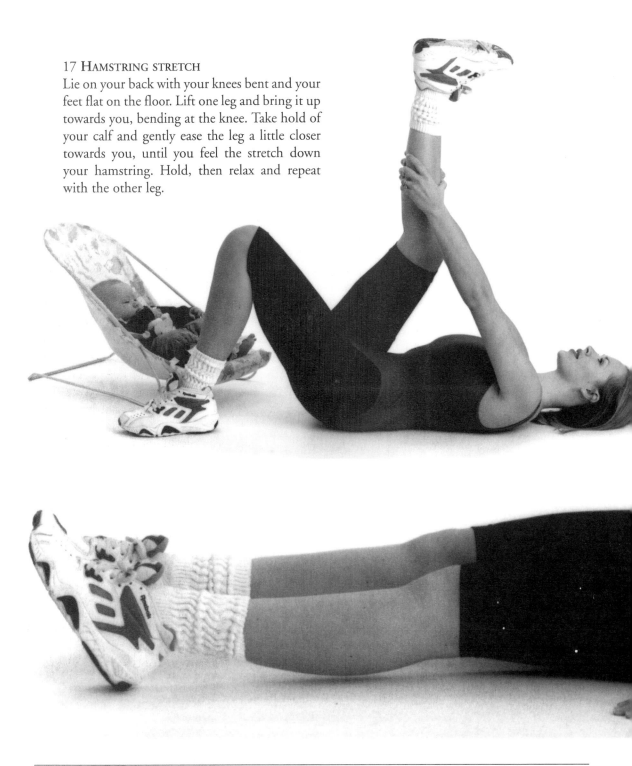

18 RELAXATION

Your baby will be fully alert by this stage and not sleeping as much as he did in the first week. Constantly caring for the new arrival and the inevitable sleepless nights may well be taking their toll by now, so relax whenever you get the chance. Forget the chores, take the phone off the hook and lie flat on your back, perhaps with a pillow under your head and your feet raised to make yourself more comfortable. Follow the same relaxation techniques as before (see Chapters 3, 5 and 6), and why not let yourself doze off?

After all, you have finished your workout!

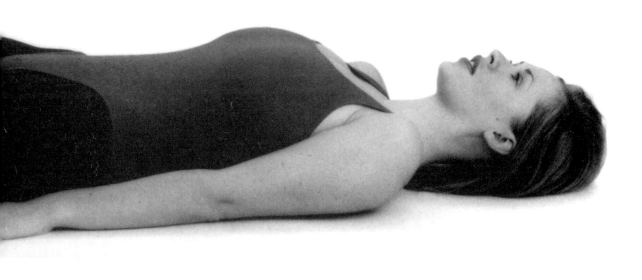

CHAPTER NINE

EXERCISE
FOR YOUR
BABY

❖

The First Six Months

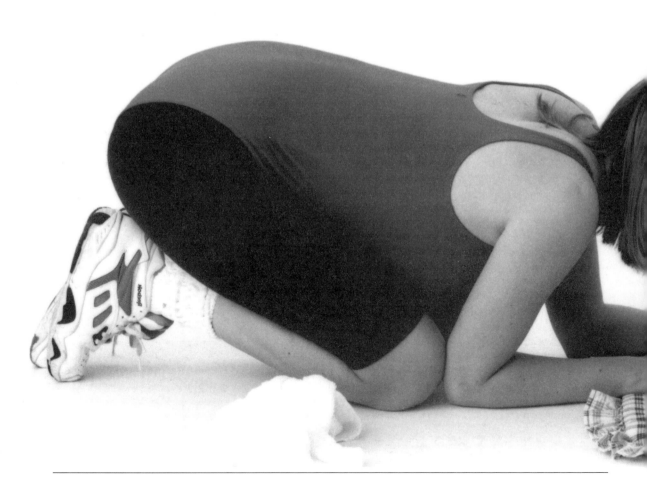

NOW THAT YOUR BABY has been born, you have another person's fitness to think about! In a few years' time she will start making her own decisions of course, but why not set her on the right track now by showing her what fun exercise can be? You are her role model, and as she grows up she will want to do everything and anything that you do – so including her in swimming, walking, cycling, workouts and so on will stimulate her interest.

From six weeks on, your baby's physical development begins to speed up. Every baby develops at her own rate, though, so do not be upset if your baby does not seem to be doing all the things that your friends' babies are – this is no reflection of her future capabilities, and she will get there in the end.

HOW YOUR BABY DEVELOPS

For the first few months of her life, your baby will obviously not be able to sit up or crawl around to play, but that does not mean she is not learning now, or is less able to join in a game.

At eight weeks old she will be able to grasp toys such as a rattle and shake it, following the noise with her eyes. This helps her to establish a relationship between what her hands are doing and what happens as a result. This is the first step towards hand-eye co-ordination – a must for most sports!

By 12 weeks she will try to swipe at any object she is shown and perhaps look from her hand to the object and back again. She will have control of her own head by now, so you will only need to support it when you pick her up or move her unexpectedly. She will have 'uncurled' from the typical round baby posture now too, and will look like she is enjoying learning how to use her body by kicking and waving at you.

At four months her hands will be under control and she will frequently be 'measuring' the distance between objects and her hand. She will be able to play 'peekaboo' games now too, by pulling her own clothes over her face. By now she should also be able to hold her head up clear of the floor when she is laid on her tummy, and being pulled up to sitting will become a favourite game as she grows stronger.

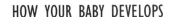

By five months she will be able to lift her head and shoulders off the ground when she is lying on her back. She is on her way to sitting by herself and will enjoy being propped up to see what is going on.

At six months some babies have already mastered crawling, but many do not until they are ten months old, and some go straight from sitting to walking without ever crawling at all. Do not rush your baby: she will find her own way of doing things in her own time.

TOYS THAT HELP

At this early age, toys do not need to be clever or complex, but it helps if they are well designed, and by people who know about what makes babies tick.

The best toys will offer a variety of things to discover and learn from, such as different weights, textures, sounds and shapes. Choose toys made by manufacturers that are established, trusted names and you will not go far wrong. It is tempting to opt for pretty pastels when you are choosing toys for a baby, but bright, primary colours are more stimulating and interesting for them and, in fact, very young babies can see black and white far better. This is why some mobiles now have colours on one side and black and white on the other, so that they are visually stimulating when babies are very young and as they grow older.

Activity centres such as this one (below) are ideal for encouraging your baby not only to develop her hand-eye co-ordination, but also to kick and swipe at the playthings hanging from it. Most babies are happy to play under a 'gym' like this for minutes at a time, fascinated by everything going on. Look for designs with detachable toys to extend their play value even further.

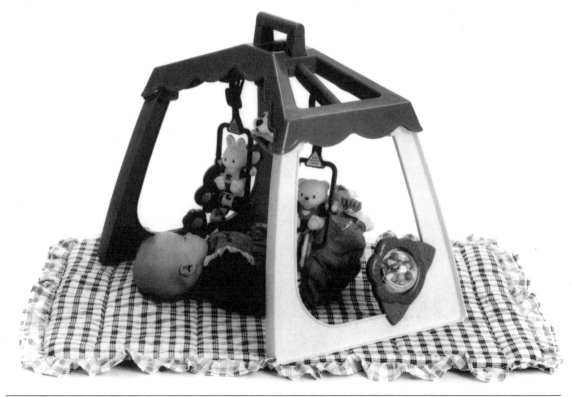

Do not forget, however, that everything is new to your baby, and what appears to you to be a plain old spoon, appears to your baby to be a wonderfully smooth and shiny plaything that is well worth a closer look. Look around your home with a baby's eye and you are sure to find plenty of suitable 'playthings' – without spending anything!

WATER BABIES

The earlier you can introduce your baby to water the better. Swimming is a wonderful exercise, and something the whole family can enjoy together, so why not start teaching her as soon as you can?

Rattles, rings, cuddly and squeaky toys and balls which your baby can hold will all help to introduce her to a wide range of textures, sounds and shapes. Playing with small toys that she can eventually pass from hand to hand will develop her hand-eye co-ordination, and she will enjoy exploring them with her mouth as well as her hands and feet. Each leg of this cuddly octopus has a different texture or makes a new noise.

It is advisable to wait until after your baby's first set of vaccinations has been completed, at around four months old, before you take her, and then choose a time when she would normally be alert and happy.

Dress her in a snug swimming costume without a nappy. Babies rarely poo in water, but if she does, get out straightaway – the costume should contain most of the damage! Find a swimming pool with a special baby pool; it will be several degrees warmer than the main pool and should be less crowded, too. Do not stay in too long – it will all be a bit strange for her at first, so ten minutes is ample.

Hold her steady in the water close to you, so you are facing one another, and smile and talk to her to reassure her. Just let her get used to the feel of the water. When you think she is ready, try holding on to her and walking in the water, encouraging her to kick with her legs and arms. Let her get used to the water splashing slightly. Do not walk backwards or on your knees, as you may fall over.

Over the course of a few sessions she will gain confidence and you will be able to play and bob about more.

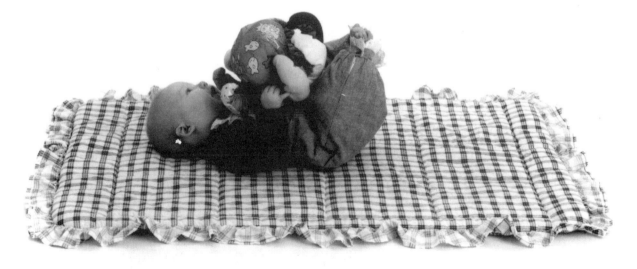

THE BABY WORKOUT

Your baby will get plenty of exercise by simply being left on a mat or towel to kick and wave. Giving her something to look at above her will keep her happy for longer, but it need not be anything fancy – the leaves in a tree are enough to fascinate a baby.

That said, there are also ways of encouraging your baby's natural progress with some gentle exercises. They are supposed to be fun for her, so never persist if she does not seem to be enjoying herself. Make the exercises part of your usual playtime together.

1 HEAD MOVEMENTS

Encourage your baby to move her head from side to side. Dangle a bright rattle above her head, then slowly move it in an arc, about 20–30cm (8–12in) from her face, waiting for her eyes and head to follow. If she loses interest, try rattling it again. Once she has moved her head one way, move the rattle to the opposite side and try again.

You do not need to have a rattle to hand to practise this: just moving your head from side to side, talking and smiling as you do so, will encourage her to follow your eyes.

When your baby is about three months old, you can encourage her to start rolling over by repeating the same exercise.

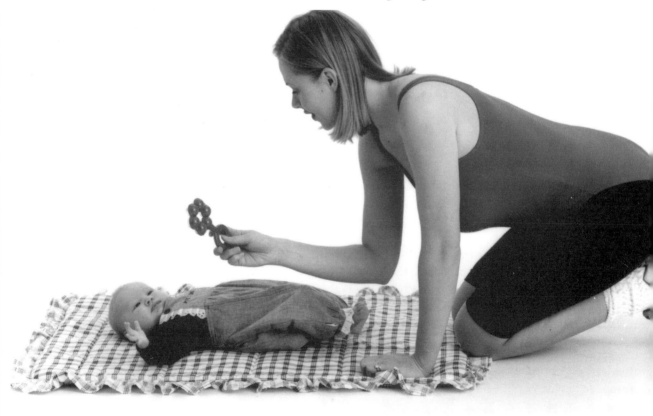

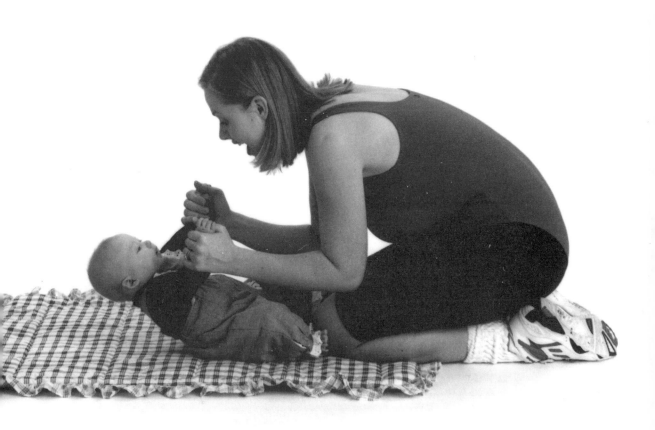

2 DEVELOPING HEAD CONTROL

This exercise strengthens your baby's neck muscles in preparation for sitting. Lie her on the floor on her back and kneel down in front of her. (If your baby is less than three months old, and small enough, sit down with your knees bent, your feet flat on the floor and rest your baby along your thighs with her head at your knees.) Talking and smiling at her, put your thumbs into her palms and wrap your fingers around the back of her hands. Turn her palms into one another, then straighten her elbows and start to lift her head and upper body gently towards you. Her head should lift in line with her shoulders, with her back straight.

Only take her as far as she can go while keeping her head controlled and in line with her body, then lower her gently down again.

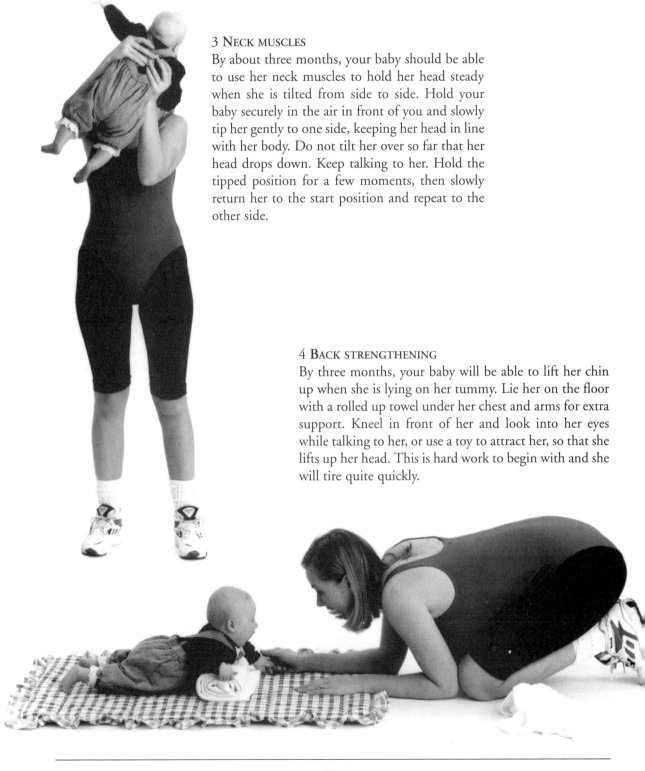

3 NECK MUSCLES

By about three months, your baby should be able to use her neck muscles to hold her head steady when she is tilted from side to side. Hold your baby securely in the air in front of you and slowly tip her gently to one side, keeping her head in line with her body. Do not tilt her over so far that her head drops down. Keep talking to her. Hold the tipped position for a few moments, then slowly return her to the start position and repeat to the other side.

4 BACK STRENGTHENING

By three months, your baby will be able to lift her chin up when she is lying on her tummy. Lie her on the floor with a rolled up towel under her chest and arms for extra support. Kneel in front of her and look into her eyes while talking to her, or use a toy to attract her, so that she lifts up her head. This is hard work to begin with and she will tire quite quickly.

INDEX

Page numbers in *italic* refer to the illustrations